FINDINGS FROM TWO DECADES OF FAMILY PLANNING RESEARCH

JOHN A. ROSS / ELIZABETH FRANKENBERG

THE POPULATION COUNCIL / NEW YORK

1993

The Population Council
1 Dag Hammarskjold Plaza
New York, New York 10017

Cover design: Diana Hrisinko

ISBN: 0-87834-078-5

Library of Congress Catalog Number 93-086577

Copyright© 1993 by The Population Council, Inc.

Any part of this volume may be copied or adapted to meet local needs without permission from the authors or the Population Council, provided that the parts copied are distributed free or at cost (not for profit). Any commercial reproduction requires prior permission from the Population Council. The authors would appreciate receiving a copy of any materials in which the text or tables from the volume are used.

Table of Contents

Foreword — v

FERTILITY, CONTRACEPTION, PROGRAMS

1. Prevalence of Contraceptive Use and Fertility Patterns — 1
2. Large-Scale Family Planning Programs — 13

PROGRAM APPROACHES

3. Community-Based Distribution — 22
4. Contraceptive Social Marketing — 27
5. Postpartum Programs — 34
6. Charges and Payments Associated with Family Planning Services — 40

METHODS

7. Contraceptive Continuation and Effectiveness — 48
8. Sterilization — 57
9. Induced Abortion — 63

RELATIONSHIP BETWEEN HEALTH AND CONTRACEPTION

10. Contraception, Fertility Patterns, and Infant/Child Mortality — 75
11. Contraceptive Use and Maternal Morbidity/Mortality — 82
12. Contraceptive Use and Health — 90

Index — 97

Foreword

We present here a selection of empirical conclusions, or findings, from the body of family planning research that has accumulated over the last two decades. Twelve topics of current interest are reviewed, as a sequel to three similar publications* issued in 1971, 1972, and 1974.

A "Findings" document compresses what has been learned into straightforward declarative statements, giving summary evidence to support each statement. In cases where a conclusion is quite well founded, with extensive supporting evidence, only illustrative or summary references are needed. In other cases citations are required for individual studies. Generalizations that are unsupported or too ambiguous to permit a definite statement do not qualify for inclusion. Methodology and theory are not the primary concern; the focus is on research results that merit particular attention.

Thus, we have identified reasonably solid conclusions, arranged them in this compact format, and listed the important evidence. The decision as to what does and does not constitute a finding is necessarily judgmental. Moreover, not all of the findings reported here are substantiated to the same degree; some are especially tenuous, and many will change as additional evidence appears. Much of the evidence is uneven, and many findings are derived from studies in only a few locations, so readers should generalize only with caution.

Twenty years ago the first "Findings" report was introduced, for reasons that remain true today. As new workers enter the field they encounter an oral tradition consisting of mixed opinions, prejudices, and information. Lacking a concise compilation of empirical results, the newcomer faces a plethora of material of varying quality, too much ever to be fully absorbed. Furthermore, conclusions that seemed certain a few years ago have undergone a shifting base of support as past studies have been forgotten, rejected, and supplanted. It has seemed important, therefore, to establish a record outlining evidence that indeed underlies each finding, with identification of which country or region it comes from. With time, this record should evolve, and then the current compilation will serve as a point of departure for restatement.

The 12 chapters fall naturally into four groups. The first two chapters, Prevalence of Contraceptive Use and Fertility Patterns, and Large-Scale Family Planning Programs, give an overall view of the massive changes that have occurred in reproductive behavior and in the organized programs designed to service and encourage them. The next four chapters follow naturally, to present approaches taken by the programs: Community-Based Distribution; Contraceptive Social Marketing; Postpartum Programs; and Charges and Payments. These chapters deal with prominent features in the extension of services to different publics. The matter of charges, and cost recovery in general, has received increasing attention and is an issue for the first three types of programs. All four chapters concern program approaches for which considerable experience has accumulated and extensive data are available. The next three chapters, Contraceptive Continuation and Effectiveness; Sterilization; and Induced Abortion, relate to specific birth-control methods. Contraception, including sterilization, has produced most of the historic fertility decline throughout the developing world, but all contraceptive methods carry some risk of failure, and abortion is often used as a back-up method or, more often, as a separate recourse. Septic abortion is a leading public health problem, one that is responsible for a large percentage of maternal deaths in the developing world. The final three chapters, Contraception, Fertility Patterns, and Infant/Child Mortality; Contraceptive Use and Maternal Morbidity/Mortality; and Contraceptive Use and Health, pertain to the health advantages of contraceptive methods, as well as to the risks they may carry.

Numerous topics are necessarily omitted as separate chapters, either because they are of less current interest or because they lack a solid body of empirical evidence that permits clear conclusions. Many of these are of considerable importance, and some are treated partially within the various chapters. As studies accumulate more can be said about some, though probably not all, of the following: the role of men; program approaches adapted to unmet needs of various types; the cost-effectiveness of program variations; mass media approaches; the rela-

---

* The three publications are: Forrest, J. E. 1971. "Postpartum services in family planning: Findings to date." *Reports on Population/Family Planning* No. 8, July 1971; Ross, J. A., A. Germain, J. E. Forrest, and J. Van Ginneken. 1972. "Findings from family planning research." *Reports on Population/Family Planning* No. 12, October 1972; and Marckwardt, A. M. 1974. "Findings from family planning research: Latin American supplement." *Reports on Population/Family Planning* No. 12, June 1974.

tive importance of different components of the quality of programs; strategies that combine family planning and health offerings; the effects of ideological positions, including religious ones, on family planning or the use of particular methods; contraceptive use among the young and unmarried; and the role of condoms which, though little used in the developing world, have gained prominence for their relation to AIDS prevention.

During the three-year gestation of this book, colleagues both at the Population Council and elsewhere have generously critiqued parts or all of the manuscript. We thank each one, and exempt all from the shortcomings that surely remain. Helpful suggestions, many of them extensive, were made by: John Bongaarts, Rodolfo Bulatao, George Cernada, John Cleland, James Foreit, Tomas Frejka, Martin Gorosh, Barbara Ibrahim, Stephen Isaacs, Cynthia Lloyd, W. Parker Mauldin, Barbara Mensch, Vincent Miller, Axel Mundigo, Naomi Rutenberg, Irving Sivin, John Stover, John Townsend, Ricardo Vernon, Mary Beth Weinberger, and Beverly Winikoff.

We express special appreciation to Nina Schwalbe for management of the many drafts of the manuscript and for improvements to the technical quality of numerous sections. We are grateful to Julie Reich for her insightful editing of these rather unusual materials, and to Sue Rosenthal and Suzanne Antonelli for final manuscript preparation. Our thanks go also to Susan Rowe and Lauren Lam for the exceptional quality of their secretarial assistance.

Partial funding for the project was provided by the United Nations Population Fund and by the Rockefeller Foundation; without this assistance the volume could not have appeared in its present form.

Chapter 1

PREVALENCE OF CONTRACEPTIVE USE AND FERTILITY PATTERNS

A transformation in contraceptive use comes from changed individual behavior, but it also reflects *societal* changes. These include new norms, a new climate of public opinion, and new infrastructures for services and supplies. Profound modifications in reproductive processes occur, which produce smaller family sizes and lower fertility rates. However, these changes move unevenly through the society, and they have moved quite unevenly through the developing world as a whole.

PREVALENCE

1. Over the last 25 to 30 years, contraceptive use has risen from about 10 percent to about 50 percent of all couples in the developing world (United Nations, 1989). Over the same period the total fertility rate (TFR) has fallen from 6.1 to 3.9 births per woman (United Nations, 1991). These changes constitute a profound transformation of childbearing patterns (see *Figures 1 and 2*).

   1.a. However, geographic patterns vary. Among the 10 largest developing countries, two have high prevalence levels, of 60 percent or more couples using a method: China (72 percent) and Brazil (66 percent). Five countries have intermediate levels of use, at about 35–55 percent: Mexico (53 percent), Indonesia (49 percent), India (43 percent), Bangladesh (39 percent), Vietnam (53 percent), and the Philippines (34 percent). Two others are at about 10 percent: Pakistan (12 percent) and Nigeria (8 percent). Certain other countries of substantial size also have very low levels of contraceptive use, probably below 10 percent: These include Sudan, Zaire, Ethiopia, and Myanmar (Ross et al., 1992; Mauldin and Segal, 1988).

   1.b. Most *countries* have low levels of contraceptive prevalence, but most *people* live in countries with moderate to high prevalence.
   Figure 3 gives the distribution of 107 countries by level of contraceptive prevalence. As it shows, almost half (48 percent) of all countries are below 30 percent prevalence, and more than two-thirds (68 percent) are below 50 percent prevalence. On the other hand, low-prevalence countries are generally the smaller ones, and most people (80 percent) live in countries where prevalence is above 30 percent.

   1.c. Sustained increases in prevalence, exceeding two percentage points per year over 10–11 years, have been registered in seven countries (bringing levels up to 48–72 percent using, depending upon the country). (All prevalence levels were measured between two or more national surveys.) The seven countries are: El Salvador, Mexico, Colombia, Hong Kong, South Korea, Indonesia, and Sri Lanka. Two other countries have experienced similar increases over a period of 5–7 years. They are Morocco and Tunisia, whose contraceptive prevalence levels have risen to 36 and 41 percent, respectively. The most rapid pace registered, a 3.1 percentage point gain per year over 10 years from 1975 to 1985, occurred in South Korea (United Nations, 1989, Table 4.) The path of increase in prevalence for numerous countries appears in *Figure 4*.

   1.d. The geographic pattern of the TFR is also uneven: The regional differences parallel those for contraceptive use. The TFR, which was high and uniform across regions in the early 1960s, is now quite uneven. Only East Asia's is near replacement, at 2.4. Other regions' TFRs are higher: Latin America's is 3.6, South Asia's is 4.4, the Middle East/North Africa's is 5.1, and sub-Saharan Africa's is still 6.6, nearly the same as in 1960–65.

   1.e. Even for the largest countries, the picture is mixed. While prevalence is already high in China and Brazil, other large countries have room for further increases. Remarkably, India alone contains 26 percent of all the new contraceptors needed to reach replacement fertility in the developing world, whereas the next few countries contain fewer than 8 percent each (*Table 1*).

   1.f. As some countries approach ceiling levels of prevalence (about 75 percent), future increases must come progressively more from countries with lower prevalence levels, less favored social settings, and weaker family planning programs. These factors may retard the pace of increases in prevalence.

Figure 1 Contraceptive prevalence trends in the developing world, by region

Percentage using contraception

Region	1960–65	1990
Total	14	51
East Asia	17	74
Latin America	11	60
South Asia	15	43
Middle East & North Africa	2	38
Sub-Saharan Africa	5	12

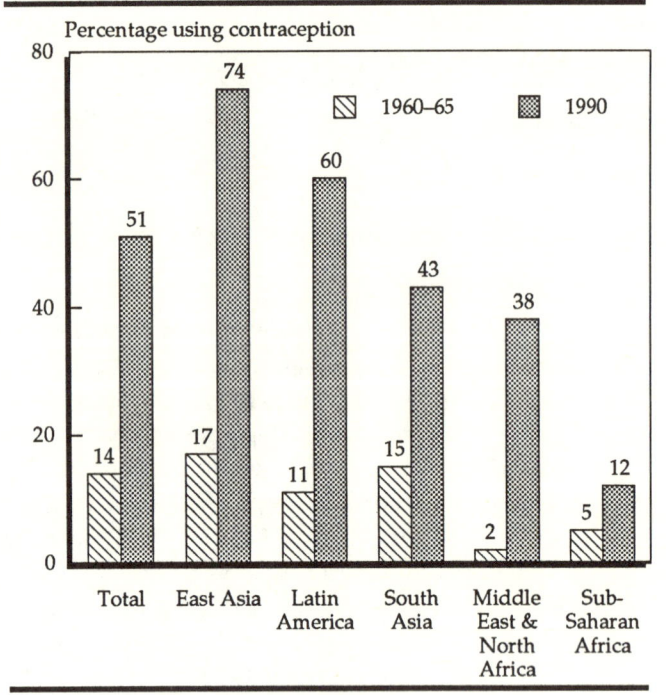

Source: Population Council Databank, 1993.

1.g. Furthermore, if prevalence is to continue to rise, use rates must increase enough to more than compensate for increasing numbers of women entering the childbearing ages. For example, to meet the United Nations medium fertility projections for the year 2000 would require 54 million more users if the base population of couples remained at its present level. But the population will grow by 30 percent from 1987 to the year 2000, requiring an additional 114 million users, or 168 million users altogether, to meet the projections.

Relation to Fertility

2. The fertility level corresponds closely to the proportion of couples using contraception. *Figure 5* shows the pattern across both developing and developed countries. Most countries lie within a narrow band of one child on either side of the line. Thus, for general purposes, changes in contraceptive prevalence and fertility can be related: A 15-point increase in contraceptive prevalence implies that the total fertility rate may fall by about one child.

Prevalence by Method

3. Three contraceptive methods, sterilization, the pill, and the IUD, account for 81 percent of all contraceptive use in the developing world.

   3.a. The remainder is due to use of the condom (6 percent) and various traditional methods (11 percent). The injectable accounts for only 2 percent of all users (*Table 2*), although its use appears to be increasing in certain countries.

   3.b. Sterilization is used by 44 percent of all couples who currently practice contraception. This percent-

Figure 2 Fertility trends in the developing world, by region

Total fertility rate

Region	1960–65	1985–90
Total	6.1	3.9
East Asia	5.9	2.4
Latin America	6.0	3.6
South Asia	6.0	4.4
Middle East and North Africa	6.9	5.1
Sub-Saharan Africa	6.7	6.6

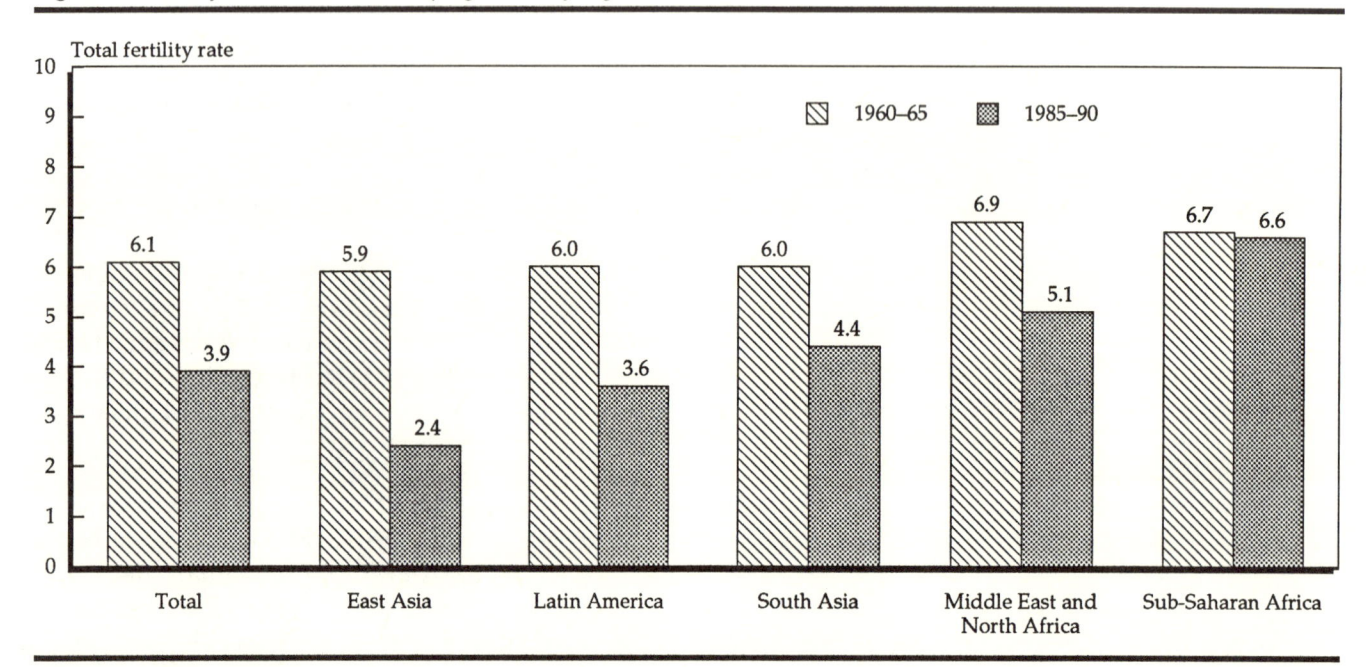

Source: United Nations, 1991.

Figure 3 Developing countries distributed by level of contraceptive prevalence

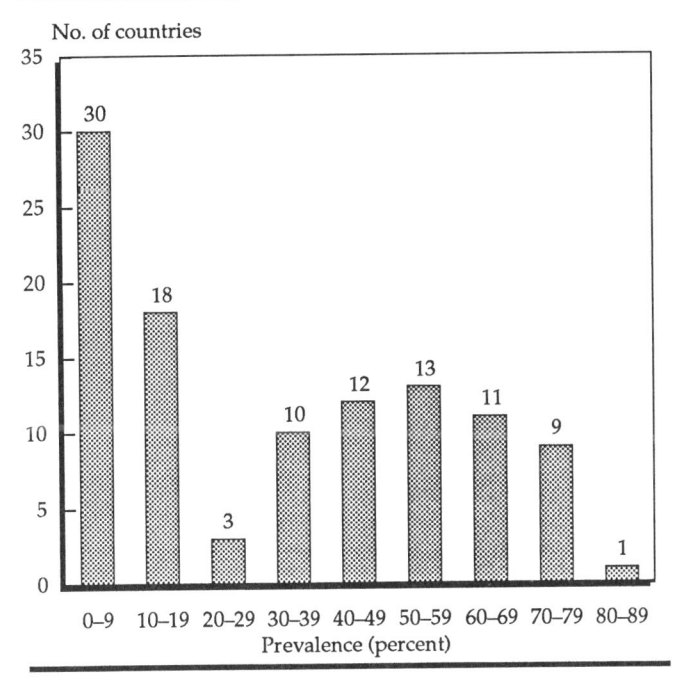

Prevalence (percent)	No. of countries
0–9	30
10–19	18
20–29	3
30–39	10
40–49	12
50–59	13
60–69	11
70–79	9
80–89	1

Source: Population Council Databank, 1993.

age reflects a gradual build-up over the past, since only small proportions undergo sterilization in any given year. That is, sterilization's *acceptance* rate is low but its *continuation* rate is high. Moreover, some build-up is due to the young ages of some adopters, as well as to the long history of the method's availability in certain countries (see Sterilization chapter).

3.c. The reverse applies to the pill: It has a high acceptance rate but a rather low continuation rate; consequently, its prevalence depends heavily upon those choosing it recently. The IUD is intermediate between the pill and sterilization in this respect.

A pattern of low continuation applies to all resupply methods and to all traditional or coitus-related methods, such as rhythm and withdrawal (which also have the highest failure rates).

3.d. The method mix for annual adoptions of contraceptives differs greatly from that for the full body of all current users. Sterilization and the IUD account for only 10 percent and 21 percent, respectively, of each year's adoptions; on the other hand they account for about three-fourths of all current users, due to their accumulation over the years. Resupply methods (the pill, injectables, and condoms) do not accumulate, and they account for a full 69 percent of the clients seen each year (traditional methods excluded; see United Nations Population Fund, 1991, Tables III.2 and III.4).

4. **Countries and regions vary widely in their method mixes and in the number of methods they make available. Those that offer several method choices have medium to high levels of contraceptive prevalence; others have lower levels (Jain, 1989; Lapham and Mauldin, 1985).**

4.a. China is exceptional in the prominent role played by the IUD: 30 percent of couples (42 percent of users) rely on it, compared to only 11 percent of users in all other LDCs. China is also unusual regarding sterilization: 36 percent of couples (50 percent of users) rely on it, and 22 percent of those currently using sterilization are men. Further, the large province of Sichuan, where the new "no scalpel" vasectomy technique was developed, accounts for one-sixth (17 percent) of all male sterilizations in the country (see Sterilization chapter). In Sichuan province, in 1984, 71 percent of new sterilizations were for men, vs. 20 percent for all China (Ross, 1991; Ross et al., 1992).

4.b. In the two most populous regions, East Asia (mainly China) and South Asia (largely India), half of all users currently rely upon sterilization (*Table 2*). These two regions differ in other respects, however; only 11 percent of users in South Asia (vs. 40 percent in East Asia) use the IUD; 15 percent (vs. 5 percent) use the hormonal methods of the pill and injectables; and 17 percent (vs. 3 percent) use such "other" methods as the condom, rhythm, and withdrawal.

Table 1 Differences between number of contraceptive users and number needed for replacement fertility

Country	# MWRA 1990 (000)	75% of MWRA (000)	# users 1990 (000)	Difference (000)	% distribution of differences
1. India	144,091	63,400	108,068	44,668	25.9
2. Nigeria	18,001	13,501	1,315	12,186	7.1
3. Pakistan	18,816	14,112	2,239	11,873	6.9
4. Bangladesh	22,041	16,531	7,262	9,269	5.4
5. Indonesia	33,026	24,770	17,249	7,521	4.4
6. Ethiopia	8,495	6,371	323	6,049	3.5
7. Iran	9,053	6,789	2,786	4,004	2.3
8. Zaire	6,457	4,843	917	3,926	2.3
9. Tanzania	4,739	3,554	142	3,412	2.0
10. Uganda	4,506	3,379	221	3,159	1.8
11. Egypt	8,982	6,736	3,666	3,070	1.8
12. Sudan	4,280	3,210	145	3,064	1.8
13. Mexico	14,682	11,012	8,507	2,505	1.5
14. Philippines	9,290	6,968	4,541	2,427	1.4
15. Afghanistan	3,148	2,361	50	2,311	1.3
16. Nepal	3,771	2,828	684	2,144	1.2
17. Kenya	4,313	3,235	1,224	2,011	1.2
18. Ghana	3,259	2,444	437	2,007	1.2
19. Mozambique	2,699	2,025	27	1,998	1.2
20. Vietnam	10,030	7,522	5,655	1,867	1.1
83 other countries	—	—	—	—	24.7
Total	—	—	—	—	100.0

Source: Ross et al., 1992.

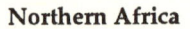

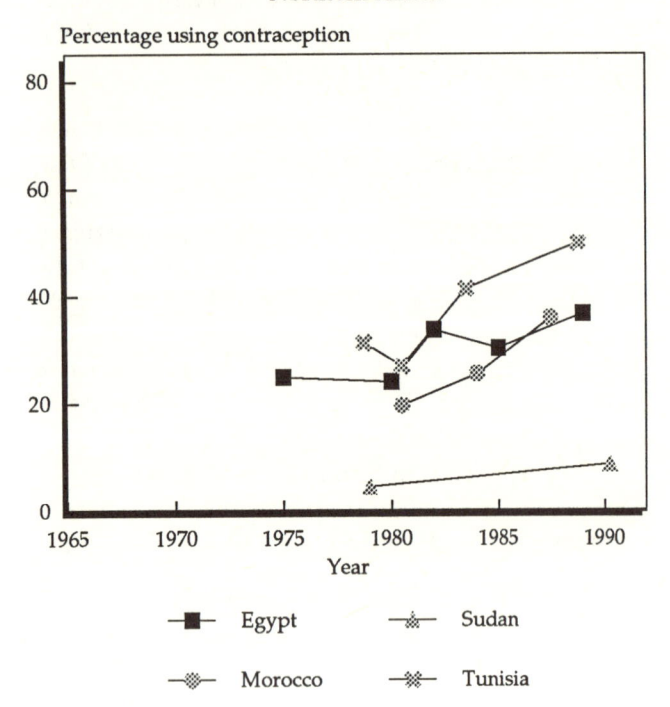

Figure 4 Trends in the percentage of married women of childbearing age currently using contraception, developing regions

Northern Africa
- Egypt
- Sudan
- Morocco
- Tunisia

Sub-Saharan Africa
- Botswana
- Nigeria
- Ghana
- Senegal
- Kenya
- Sudan (North)
- Mauritius
- Zimbabwe

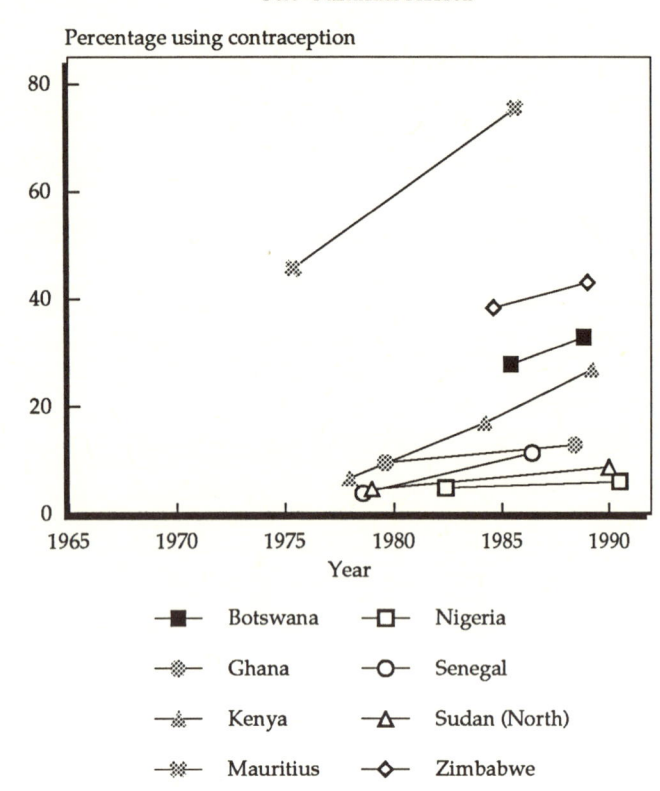

Eastern and Western Asia
- China
- Rep. of Korea
- Hong Kong
- Turkey
- Jordan

South Asia
- Bangladesh
- Pakistan
- India
- Sri Lanka
- Nepal

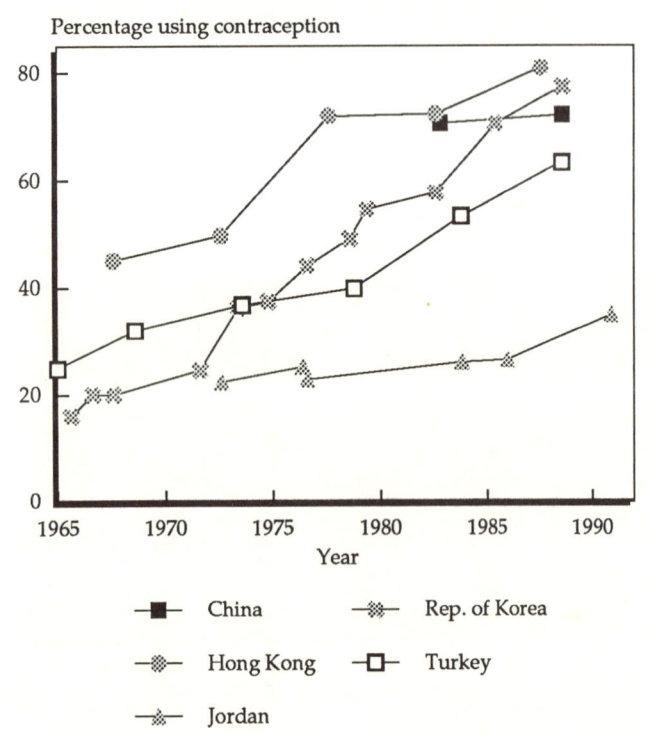

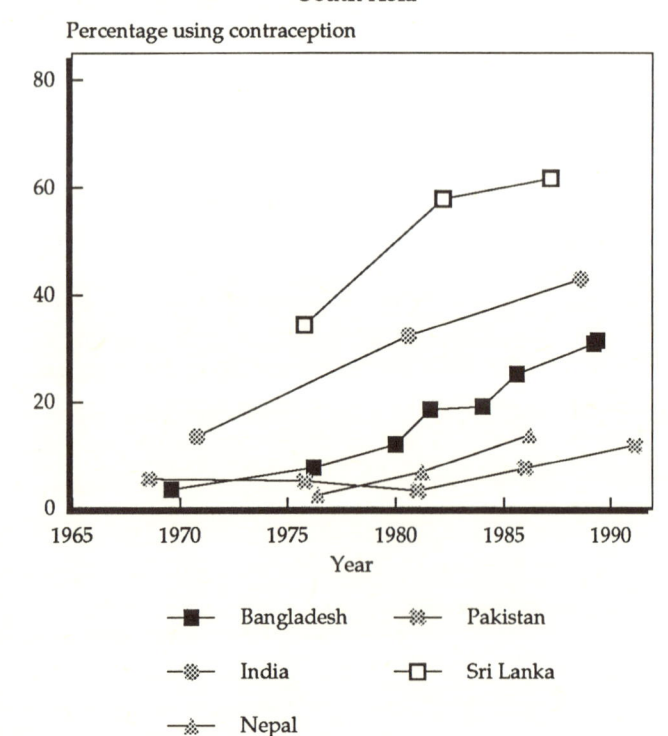

Figure 4 (continued)

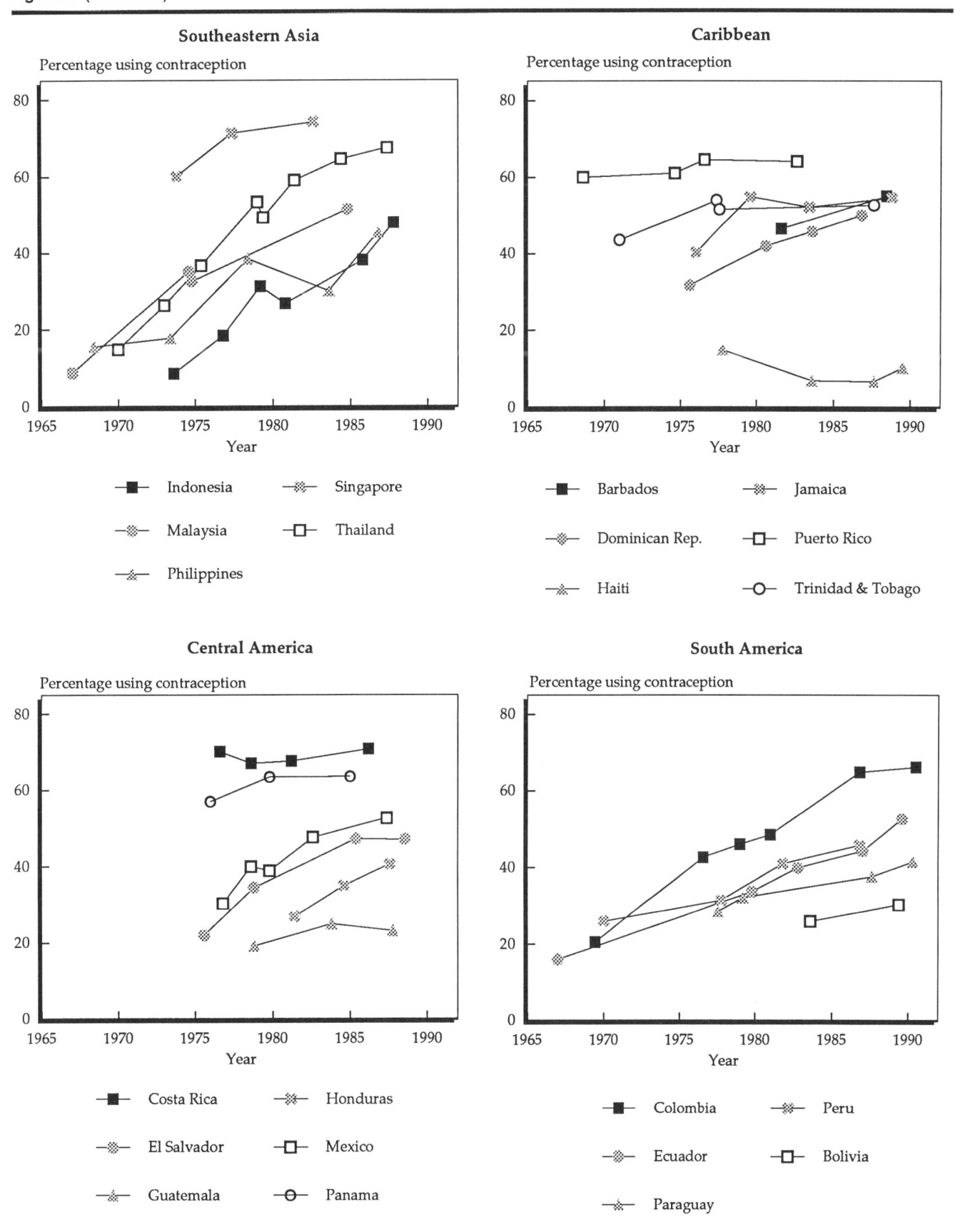

Southeastern Asia

Percentage using contraception

- ■ Indonesia
- ※ Singapore
- ※ Malaysia
- □ Thailand
- ※ Philippines

Caribbean

Percentage using contraception

- ■ Barbados
- ※ Jamaica
- ※ Dominican Rep.
- □ Puerto Rico
- ※ Haiti
- ○ Trinidad & Tobago

Central America

Percentage using contraception

- ■ Costa Rica
- ※ Honduras
- ※ El Salvador
- □ Mexico
- ※ Guatemala
- ○ Panama

South America

Percentage using contraception

- ■ Colombia
- ※ Peru
- ※ Ecuador
- □ Bolivia
- ※ Paraguay

Source: Weinberger, 1991, Figure 2, p. 565–566.

Figure 5 Contraceptive prevalence and total fertility rate, developing and developed countries, 1993

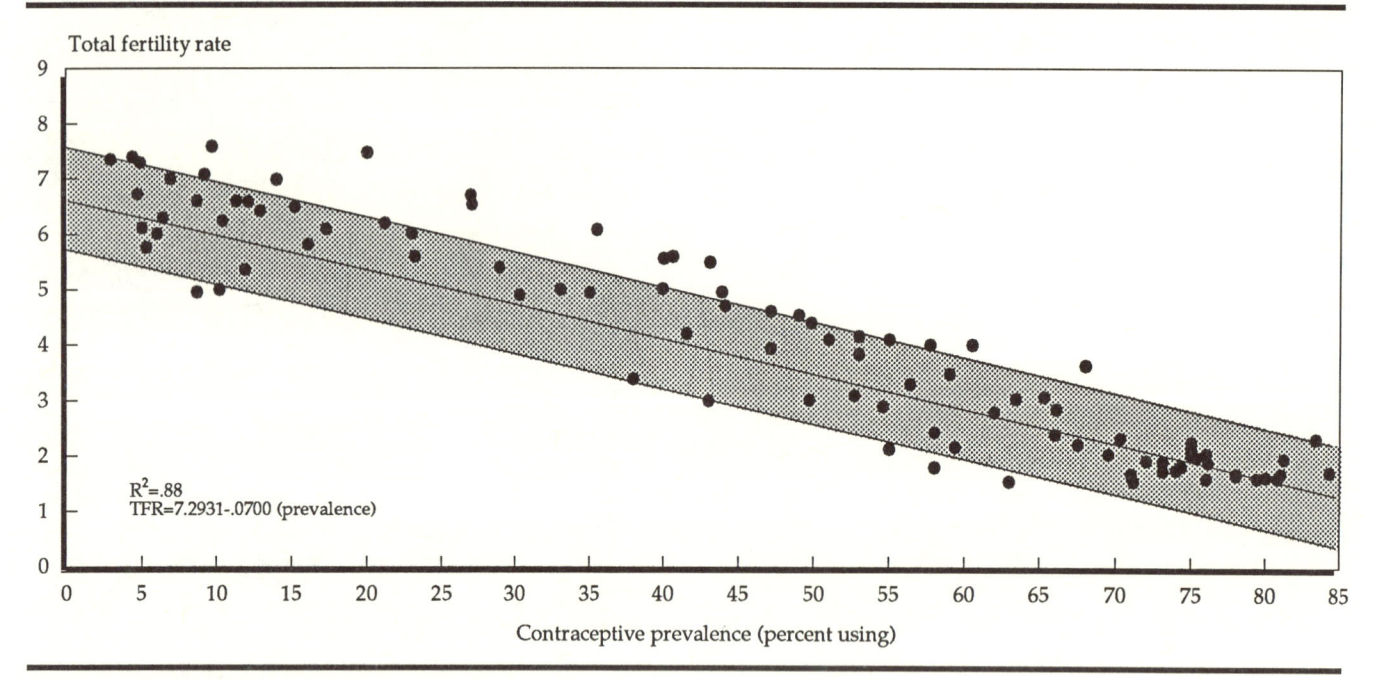

[Scatter plot: Total fertility rate (y-axis, 0-9) vs. Contraceptive prevalence (percent using) (x-axis, 0-85). R² = .88; TFR = 7.2931 − .0700 (prevalence). The shaded area is +/− one child from the regression line.]

Source: Population Council Databank, 1993.

4.c. The Latin American method mix is similar to that of South Asia, except that there is less sterilization use and more pill use. The other two regions are quite different: In sub-Saharan Africa and North Africa/Middle East the overall proportion of couples using contraception is much smaller and those who do use rely more heavily upon traditional and folk methods ("Other" in *Table 2*) than do people in other regions.

5. **Historically, as the overall prevalence of contraceptive use has grown, it has done so through modern methods, which have outpaced or replaced growth in use of traditional methods.**[1]

5.a. Traditional methods are rather little used in the developing world as a whole. They involve no resupply, since they include withdrawal, rhythm, abstinence for contraceptive intent, and "other," all as reported in national surveys. They exclude vaginals and condoms, which are classified under "modern methods"; the issue of their labelling as either traditional or modern is a minor one anyway, since use of vaginals is minimal, never exceeding 2 percent of couples in 62 of 66 countries surveyed, and use of condoms never exceeds 5 percent of couples in 56 of the 66 countries surveyed (Ross et al., 1992).

5.b. In the developing world (*Table 2*), only 11 percent of all contraceptive users rely upon traditional methods. This percentage is low partly because most users are in countries where traditional methods play a minor role, as in China and India. In two regions, sub-Saharan Africa and the Middle East/North Africa, traditional methods have a higher share of users, at 31–37 percent, but total use is low there. As a percentage of all couples, rather than users, tradi-

Table 2 Percentage distribution and number (in 000s) of contraceptive users, by method, according to region, 1990

Method	Sub-Saharan Africa %	(N)	Middle East/ North Africa %	(N)	East Asia %	(N)	South Asia %	(N)	Latin America %	(N)	Total %	(N)
Sterilization	10	1,083	5	775	49	88,429	49	63,154	36	15,860	44	169,301
Female	10	1,078	5	761	38	69,054	37	48,618	35	15,394	35	134,904
Male	0	5	0	14	11	19,466	11	14,578	1	467	9	34,529
Pill	27	2,830	33	5,191	5	9,034	11	14,869	29	12,663	12	44,587
Injectable	13	1,328	1	100	0	582	4	5,040	2	885	2	7,934
IUD	9	983	23	3,613	40	71,258	11	13,702	11	4,740	25	94,296
Condom	4	397	7	1,136	4	6,311	9	11,905	4	1,860	6	21,609
Other	37	3,901	31	4,845	3	4,751	17	21,641	18	8,024	11	43,163
Total	100	10,521	100	15,661	100	180,365	100	130,310	100	44,033	100	380,890

Source: Mauldin and Ross, 1992, p.7.

Table 3 Percent of MWRA using traditional methods over time, by region, for selected countries

Region	% using traditional methods
Latin America	
Bolivia	15–18
Colombia	11–13
Costa Rica	9–12
Ecuador	9–12
Paraguay	13–16
Peru	24–24
Asia	
Malaysia	10–31
Philippines	15–23
Sri Lanka	22–25
Middle East/North Africa	
Turkey	29–34

Note: No relevant cases in sub-Saharan Africa.
Comment: No time trend is available for Vietnam, but in its 1988 survey, 15 percent of couples were using traditional methods. In South Korea, Taiwan, and Hong Kong, traditional method use appears to have been falling, to below 10 percent of couples.
Source: Population Council Databank, 1993.

tional methods in those two regions fall below 10 percent in all 30 countries surveyed, except Mauritius, Lebanon, and Turkey (Ross et al., 1992, Table 8).

5.c. The same pattern, of rather low use of traditional methods, holds in the other two regions: It exceeds 10 percent of couples in only four of 15 Asian countries and in only seven of 21 Latin American countries. For the whole developing world use of traditional methods falls below the 10 percent level in 52 of 66 countries with national surveys; only 14 countries fall at or above it. For 10 of these 14, time trends are available, as follows.

5.d. Time trends: Traditional methods have remained important over time in certain countries, when judged as a percent of all couples using them. *Table 3* provides figures for countries with multiple surveys, where the latest survey gives 10 percent or more using. Most ranges apply to periods in the 1980s.

Prevalence by Personal Characteristics

6. **The prevalence of contraceptive use is uneven across subgroups; it has increased in certain subgroups that were historically slow to adopt a method.**

6.a. Prevalence is typically highest in the middle range of age and parity (Robey et al., 1992). Interest in contraception builds after the first and second child arrive and as the couple ages. After rising to a peak, it declines as secondary sterility sets in. Lower prevalence among older women can also reflect historical factors, as their attitudes were formed during more conservative times. Lower prevalence at the upper parities may also reflect the age factor; moreover, high parity is itself a result of low contraceptive use over the years.

6.b. The age distributions for the three principal contraceptive methods are quite similar in shape, and they overlap greatly. By mean age, sterilization users are oldest, then IUD users, and then pill users; however, the means conceal the very large overlaps in the three distributions (Population Council unpublished tabulations from national sample surveys).

6.c. Time trends show a nearly universal downward movement in the average age and parity of contraceptive users. Younger couples, with fewer children, have adopted contraception at a faster pace than have other subgroups (Ross et al., 1988; Ross, 1979). In all age groups the percentage using a method has risen; among young couples this has been encouraged by declines in desired family size.

6.d. The education pattern for contraceptive use is consistent across countries: Use rises regularly with education level (Weinberger, 1991). This is not necessarily true, however, for each contraceptive method; for example, patterns of sterilization by education are quite inconsistent across countries.

6.e. Differences in prevalence by education level tend to persist as overall prevalence rises. A comparison of WFS and DHS surveys done in the same 15 countries, roughly 10 years apart, shows rising use levels in all groups, but with a persistent education gap. Average WFS levels were 16 percent using among the uneducated and 48 percent using among those with 10 or more years of schooling. Later, in the DHS surveys, these figures rose to 31 and 58 percent, reducing the gap only from 32 to 27 percent.

However, the gap appears to diminish considerably in countries where prevalence rises to a high level, as in Thailand. In such cases, a contraceptive saturation point is reached among the highly educated, and the less educated groups move to catch up.

6.f. Paradoxically, while use is greater among the better educated, the less educated groups have been chiefly responsible for the historic increases in national prevalence levels. Their large numbers control both the level and the trend of the overall prevalence figures. (Note that younger couples tend to be better educated, which partly explains their relatively rapid uptake of contraception.)

6.g. By residence, contraceptive use is nearly always greater among urban than rural populations. Over time, use has risen almost evenly in both urban and rural sectors; thus, in many countries the gap between them has not yet narrowed. The comparison of WFS and DHS surveys for the same 15 countries as for education shows mean rural prevalence at 20 percent and urban at 36 percent in the WFS series. The subsequent DHS values were 36 percent for rural areas (the same as in the urban sector 10 years earlier) and 51 percent in urban areas, thus preserving the same differential as before (Weinberger, 1991). However, as with education, residential differences probably narrow when use among urban residents stabilizes at a high (saturation) level and use among the rural sector continues to rise.

7. **A contraceptive method that sets in motion a widespread delivery system will change the method mix.**

   7.a. Use of the pill increased sharply in Thailand when medical authorities recognized that the method lent itself to distribution throughout the rural sector by means of auxiliary nurse midwives already stationed there (see CBD chapter).

   7.b. The pill and condom can be delivered by unpaid village workers, permitting the creation of community-based programs that have vastly expanded use (especially of the pill) in numerous countries. In Indonesia the pill is delivered to roughly 35,000–50,000 service points (see CBD chapter).

FERTILITY TRENDS

As noted above and in *Figure 2*, fertility trends have been sharply downward in the developing world as a whole. This section provides details and describes geographic disparities in that overall picture.

8. **Total fertility rates have declined sharply in the regions of Asia and Latin America, but rather little in Africa (*Figure 6*).**

   8.a. Using the UN regional definitions, Northern and Southern Africa are culturally distinct, but both have experienced appreciable fertility declines. However, in Middle Africa and Western Africa, no change in fertility levels is visible (see *Figure 6*) between 1965–70 and 1985–90, and the fall is merely .13 of a child in sub-Saharan Africa as a whole. Nevertheless, DHS survey reports indicate that declines have apparently begun in Botswana, Kenya, and Zimbabwe, and perhaps in part of Nigeria.

   8.b. The largest subregional declines have occurred in East and Southeast Asia, as well as in the Caribbean and Central America.

9. **Since the mid 1960s, fertility has declined by over 25 percent in 17 of 43 developing countries, of which 19 are in Asia and the Pacific, 17 in Latin America, and 7 in Africa.**

   9.a. The total population of the seven African countries[2] with these substantial fertility declines is relatively small, about 133 million people; the bulk of sub-Saharan Africa has shown little decline. In Latin America, however, the population of countries with large fertility declines and countries with already low fertility (Argentina and Uruguay) totals more than 400 million, or about 93 percent of the population of Latin America. In Asia, 11 countries have had fertility declines of 40 percent or more, and declines of at least 25 percent have occurred in the countries there with populations over 100 million, with the exception of Pakistan (China, India, Indonesia; also Bangladesh, with a 24 percent decline). Countries with declines of 25 percent or more total over 2.5 billion people, or 84 percent of the Asia total (75 percent outside of China) (United Nations, 1991).

   9.b. The 14 countries with populations of 45 million or more experienced, in the aggregate, a decline in the TFR of 40 percent over some 15 to 20 years (late 1960s to early or late 1980s) (*Table 4*). These countries contain 78 percent of the total developing world, including China; without China the decline was 27 percent rather than 40 percent. These two declines represent 62 and 41 percent (with and without China) of the movement to replacement fertility (TFR of 2.1).

10. **For LDCs as a whole, the pace of decline diminished in the last two five-year periods,[3] as it did overall in Latin America and in Asia (see *Figure 6*).**

    10.a. The pace of decline was irregular in subregions, especially in Asia (note that East Asia, with China, Japan, and South Korea, had reached a near minimum fertility level by the 1980s and could hardly fall much further).

    10.b. Thus, the fall in the TFR diminished through 1980–85, and remained slow in 1985–90 for all LDCs, for all Latin America, and for all Asia. For subregions the decline in the TFR persisted only in Northern and Southern Africa, in the three Latin American subregions, and in three Asian subregions, again an irregular pattern. Note that the TFR in East Asia, with China, was already rather low and could not easily fall further.

Figure 6 Trends in total fertility rates, developing regions and subregions

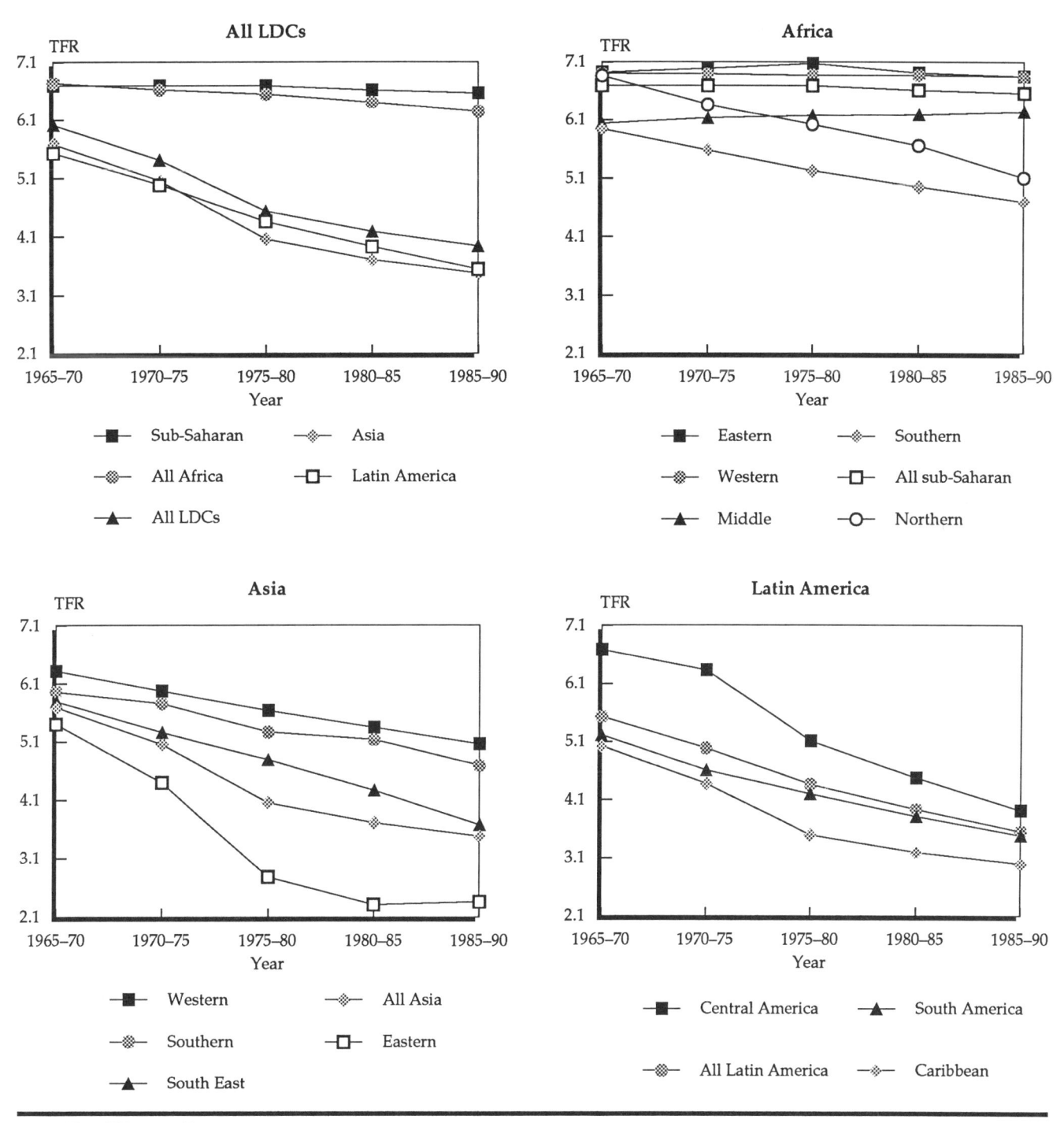

[Four line graphs showing TFR trends from 1965-70 to 1985-90 for All LDCs, Africa, Asia, and Latin America and their subregions]

Source: United Nations, 1991.

11. **Declines are less marked when the TFR is corrected for infant and child survival, and for age structures that support high crude birth rates.**

   11.a. The TFR refers strictly to live births; many newborns die shortly thereafter. Because fewer newborns have been dying in recent years, the actual number of surviving entries to the child population has not declined as much as births have. These softer declines are displayed in *Figure 7*, which shows the TFR decline along with a second line, for the net reproduction rate, which corrects for survival.[4] The decline for surviving children is not as impressive as the decline for births; the survival line is 19 percent higher (63/53) by the end of the period shown. Through

CHAPTER 1 FINDINGS 9

Table 4 Among countries with populations of 45 million or more in 1985, total fertility rates and percentage change in fertility, 1965–70 to latest data available

Country	Population size 1985 (in 000s)	Total fertility rate 1965–70*	Latest data	% change	% decline towards replacement level
Bangladesh	101,147	6.91	5.05 (1989[a])	–27	–39
Brazil	135,564	5.31	3.53 (1984 DHS)	–34	–55
China	1,059,522	5.99	2.30 (1988[a])	–62	–95
Egypt	47,578	6.56	4.38 (1988 DHS)	–33	–49
India	769,183	5.69	4.20 (1989[a])	–26	–42
Indonesia	166,464	5.57	3.30 (1987 DHS)	–41	–65
Iran	47,624	6.97	5.64 (1980–85 UN)	–19	–27
Mexico	79,376	6.70	3.80 (1986 DHS)	–43	–63
Nigeria	95,198	6.90	6.90 (1980–85 UN)	0	0
Pakistan	103,241	7.00	7.00 (1980–85 UN)	0	0
Philippines	55,120	6.04	4.74 (1980–85 UN)	–22	–33
Thailand	51,604	6.14	2.32 (1987 DHS)	–62	–95
Turkey	50,345	5.62	3.04 (1988[a])	–46	–73
Vietnam	60,059	5.94	4.06 (1988[a])	–32	–49
Total	2,822,027	6.01	3.60	–40	–62

*UN data for 1965–1970.
[a] Sources: Data for Bangladesh, China and Turkey — Population Council Data Files, 1991; India — R. Ridker, World Bank, personal communication, April 30, 1991; and Vietnam — Socialist Republic of Vietnam, National Committee for Population and Family Planning, *Vietnam Demographic and Health Survey*, Hanoi, 1990.
Source: Freedman and Blanc, 1992.
Reproduced with the permission of the Alan Guttmacher Institute from Ronald Freedman and Ann K. Blanc, "Fertility Transition: An Update," *International Family Planning Perspectives*, Volume 18, No. 2, June 1992.

time more children remain in the population than previously, so the downward trend in surviving children is not as sharp as the downward trend in births.

11.b. The *crude birth rate* (not shown) also declines less than the TFR; by 2000–2005 it is also projected to fall to only 63 percent of its 1965–1970 value. Because the CBR is based upon the total population, present age structures, which will persist for some decades, will tend to sustain high birth rates and large absolute numbers of births.

12. Fertility is unlikely to decline unless mortality has declined sufficiently to raise life expectancy to about 50 to 60 years.

12.a. With rather few exceptions, TFRs are about 6–7.5 children per woman in countries where life expectancy is below 50 years. Above 55 years, a much closer association appears, with fertility falling rather regularly with lower mortality (see *Figure 8* for 106 developing countries; updated from Bongaarts, 1986).

12.b. Certain outliers in *Figure 8* are exceptional in various respects. India and Indonesia, with strong family planning programs, have lower fertility than expected, while in a cluster of Middle Eastern countries (upper right of *Figure 8*) high fertility persists in the presence of relatively high life expectancy (these countries are Iraq, Iran, Jordan, Oman, Saudi Arabia, and Syria).

12.c. "No fertility transition has been observed to

Figure 7 Total fertility rate (TFR) and net reproduction rate (NRR): time trend for all developing countries

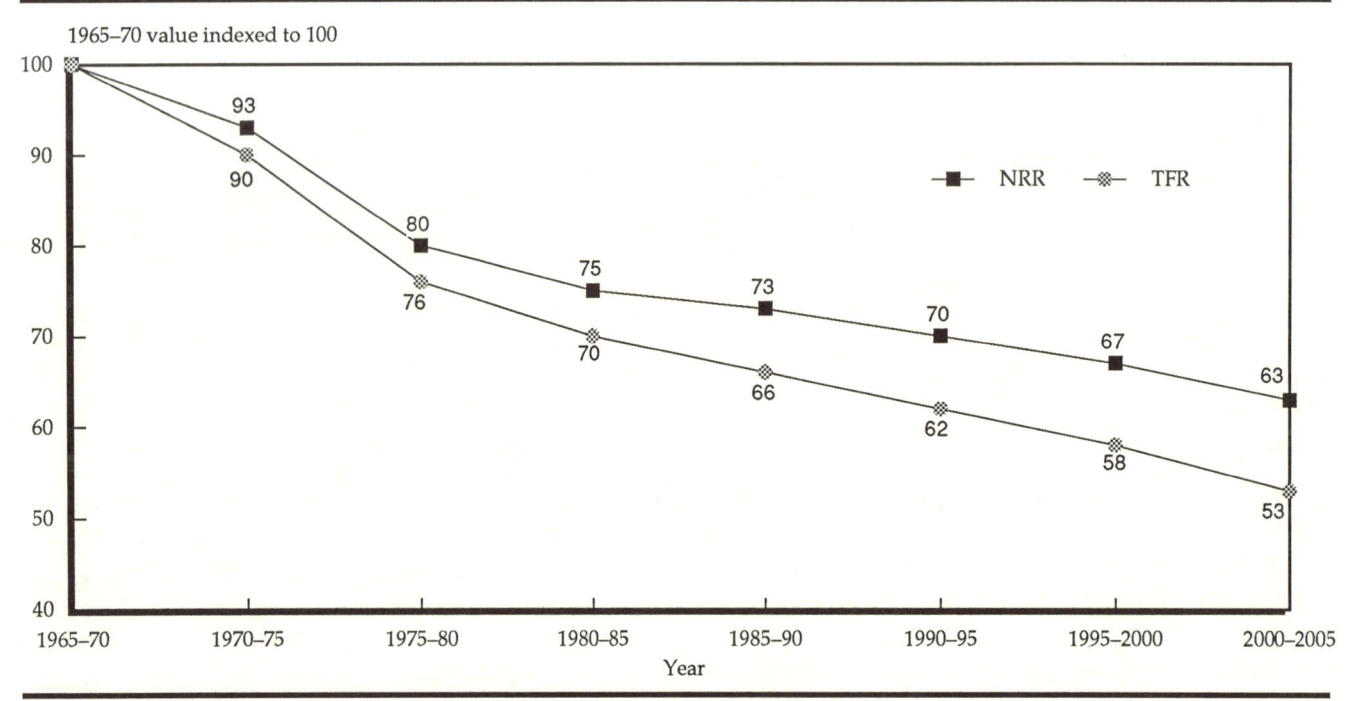

Year	NRR	TFR
1965–70	100	100
1970–75	93	90
1975–80	80	76
1980–85	75	70
1985–90	73	66
1990–95	70	62
1995–2000	67	58
2000–2005	63	53

(1965–70 value indexed to 100)

Source: United Nations, 1991.

Figure 8 Total fertility rates and life expectancies at birth for 106 developing countries (average for 1985–90 period)

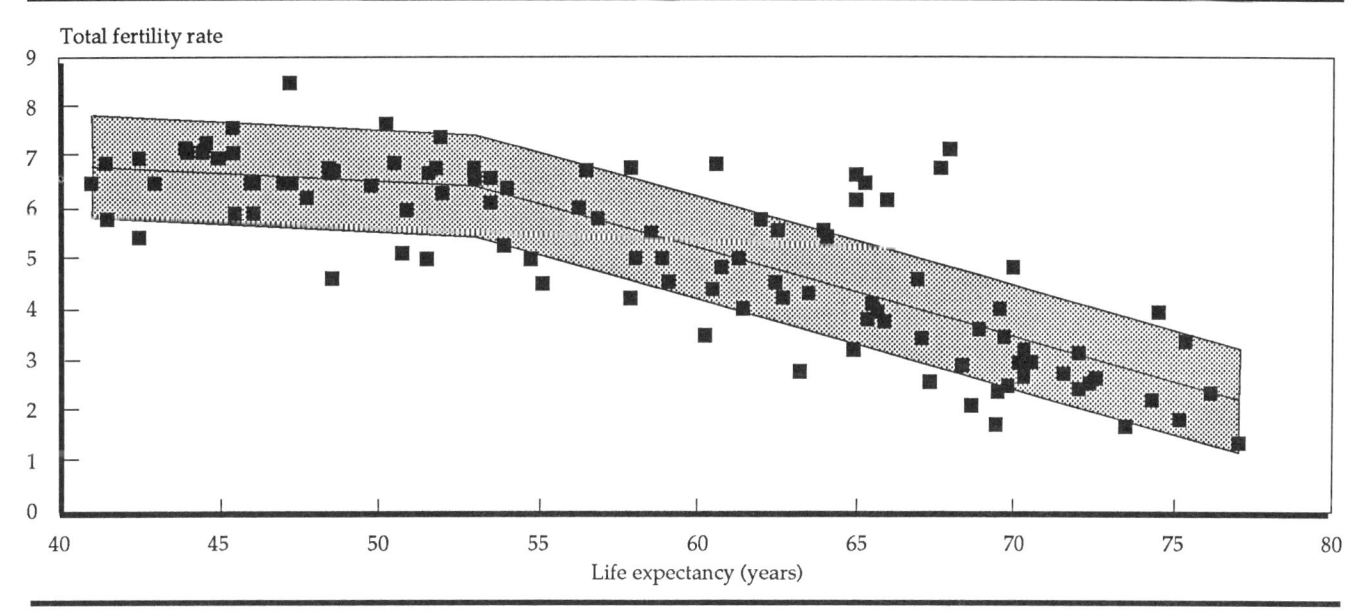

Source: United Nations, 1991.

start in any developing country until expectation of life at birth had stayed above 50 for at least five years and finally reached at least 53." Life expectancy of 53 has been in the recent past "...almost always a necessary condition for fertility transition..." and 56 a necessary condition for a rapid transition. However, those levels are not *sufficient*, since many countries lack a transition even many years after reaching them. Other factors may count, such as education, urbanization, and contraceptive availability, individually or in combination (Bulatao and Elwan, 1985).

13. **The more recent the fertility decline, the faster it has been, on average.**

    13.a. Fertility declines in some developing countries occurred considerably more rapidly than had the historic declines in Europe. Kirk's (1971) analysis, confirmed by Berelson (1978), showed that "... there has been an acceleration in the rate at which countries move through the demographic transition from high to low birth rates...the average length of time required for a country to pass through this stage...has been greatly reduced, from some 50 years for countries entering the transition in 1875–99 to half that time or less for those countries entering the transition...since 1950." (See *Table 5*)

14. **Subreplacement fertility has been reached by some developing countries and most developed countries (United Nations, 1991; Freedman and Blanc, 1992).**

    14.a. As of the 1985-90 period, Cuba, Hong Kong, Mauritius, Singapore, South Korea, and Taiwan were all below replacement (ranging from 0.65 to 0.93 surviving daughters per woman). Others were close to replacement: China at 1.11, North Korea at 1.17, and Thailand at 1.15.

    14.b. In developed countries fertility is at an all-time low: 24 of the 30 countries included in United Nations statistics were below replacement fertility in 1985–90, including the United States and all of Western Europe, except Ireland; in addition, the former USSR had an NRR of 1.11.

    14.c. Historically, low fertility has sometimes been followed by rebounds; since low fertility is generally due to voluntary and deliberate control, it is subject to reversals.

Table 5 Years historically and currently required for countries to reduce annual crude birth rates from 35 to 20

Period in which birth rate reached ≤35	Number of countries	Number of years required to reach birth rate of 20		
		Mean	Median	Range
1875–99	9	48	50	40–55
1900–24	7	38	32	24–58
1925–49	5	31	28	25–37
1950–	22	22	21	11–40

Note: First three rows from Kirk, 1971. Fourth row from Berelson, 1978, as an update of earlier estimates by Kirk and with extension from 6 to 22 countries. Both Kirk and Berelson used linear extrapolation to determine years needed to complete the crude birth rate decline to 20.
Source: Kirk, 1971; Berelson, 1978.

NOTES

1. Where overall contraceptive prevalence is high, traditional methods account for a smaller proportion of the method mix, as seen across 167 national surveys (multiple surveys in some countries over time).

Method mix by level of prevalence[a]

Method	<20	20–39	40–59	60+
Sterilization	18	19	24	33
IUD	7	13	14	9
Pill	26	33	25	25
Injectables	3	4	4	3
Condom	5	4	7	13
Vaginals	1	2	2	2
All modern	60	75	76	85
Traditional	40	25	24	15
All	100	100	100	100
(N)	(50)	(46)	(50)	(21)

[a]Figures are unweighted and therefore differ from those in Table 2. The traditional method share appears large1 because every country is given equal weight, and in many small countries the traditional methods account for much of the rather low amount of all contraceptive use.
Source: Population Council databank.

2. These countries are Algeria, Egypt, Mauritius, Morocco, Réunion, South Africa, and Tunisia.

3. Based on United Nations information; from empirical data through 1980–85, and largely from projections for 1985–90.

4. This line is for the net reproduction rate (NRR), which corrects the total fertility rate for the prevailing female mortality rates. It gives the number of daughters produced from one generation to the next under current fertility and female mortality rates. Note that some of the difference in *Figure 7* reflects survival gains after the childhood years, though these are minor.

REFERENCES

Berelson, B. 1978. "Prospects and programs for fertility reduction: What? Where? *Population and Development Review* 4(4):579–616.

Bongaarts, J. 1986. "The transition in reproductive behavior in the third world." *World Population and U.S. Policy: The Choices Ahead* (Jane Menken, Ed.). New York: W. W. Norton, Inc.

Bulatao, R. A. and Ann Elwan. 1985. "Fertility and Mortality Transition: Patterns, Projections, and Interdependence." *World Bank Staff Working Papers* No. 681, Population and Development Series No. 6.

Freedman, R. and A. K. Blanc. 1992. "Fertility transition: An update." *International Family Planning Perspectives* 18(2): 44–50.

Jain, A. K. 1989. "Fertility reduction and the quality of family planning services." *Studies in Family Planning* 20(1):1–16.

Kirk, D. 1971. "A new demographic transition?" In *Rapid Population Growth: Consequences and Policy Implications*. National Academy of Sciences, Baltimore: Johns Hopkins University Press.

Lapham, R. J. and W. P. Mauldin. 1985. "Contraceptive prevalence: The influence of organized family planning programs." *Studies in Family Planning* 16(3):117–137.

Mauldin, W.P. and S.J. Segal. 1986. *Prevalence of Contraceptive Use in Developing Countries: A Chart Book*. New York: The Rockefeller Foundation.

Mauldin, W.P. and S.J. Segal. 1988. "Prevalence of contraceptive use: Trends and issues." *Studies in Family Planning* 19(6):335–353.

Robey, B., S. O. Rutstein, and L. Morris. 1992. "National family planning surveys: What women say." *Population Reports*, Series M, No. 11, Vol. 20(4).

Ross, J.A. 1979. "Declines in the age and family size of family planning program acceptors: International trends." *Studies in Family Planning* 10(10):290–299.

———. 1991. "Sterilization: Past, Present, Future." *Population Council Working Papers* No. 29. Condensed, under same title, in *Studies in Family Planning* 23(3):187–198.

Ross, J.A., M. Rich, J.P. Molzan, M. Pensak. 1988. *Family Planning and Child Survival: 100 Developing Countries*. New York: Byrd Press.

Ross, J. A., W. P. Mauldin, S. R. Green, E. R. Cooke. 1992. *Family Planning and Child Survival Programs as Assessed in 1991*. New York: The Population Council.

United Nations. 1989. "Levels and Trends of Contraceptive Use As Assessed in 1988." *Population Studies* No. 110. ST/ESA/SER.A/110. New York: United Nations Dept. of International Economic and Social Affairs.

———. 1991. "World Population Prospects 1990." *Population Studies* No. 120, ST/ESA/SER.A/120. New York: United Nations, Dept of International Economic and Social Affairs. Sales No. E.91.XIII.4.

United Nations Population Fund. 1991. *Contraceptive Requirements and Demand for Contraceptive Commodities in Developing Countries in the 1990s*. Submitted to the UNFPA Consultative Meeting on Contraceptive Requirements in Developing Countries by the Year 2000, New York, February 25–26.

Weinberger, M.B. 1991. "Recent trends in contraceptive behavior." In *Demographic and Health Surveys World Conference: Proceedings*, Vol. 1. Columbia, Maryland: IRD/Macro International, Inc.

Chapter 2

LARGE-SCALE FAMILY PLANNING PROGRAMS

Large-scale programs to expand contraceptive use and/or reduce fertility rates now cover most of the developing world's population. However, the programs vary considerably in strength and coverage, as well as in the variety of contraceptive methods they offer. Many individual countries have weak programs, but most people live in countries having the stronger programs. China and India alone have half of the total population of the developing world (*Table 1*). The largest eight countries have two-thirds of the total, and five of these countries, containing 58 percent of the total, have strong programs. All countries after the 17th in *Table 1* claim less than one percent of the total; program strength ranges widely in these countries.

The principal functions of the programs are to provide services, information, persuasion, and legitimation; countries vary greatly in the relative emphasis they give to these aspects. They also differ in coverage of the population for each function. Some programs operate only in clinics in the larger cities; at the other extreme, some deliver a variety of services to the doorstep in the villages.

The programs use various modes of delivery (see other chapters for information on community-based distribution, social marketing, and postpartum programs).

The findings immediately following are based upon 30 ratings, or scores, of program effort as applied to approximately 100 developing countries (all those with populations of one million or more). The ratings are based upon the judgments of knowledgeable respondents for each country. The 30 scores fall into four dimensions of effort as shown in the box: policy, services, evaluation, and availability of methods. Each score, for each country, can range from zero to four, so the maximum total score is 120. Because the totals vary for the four dimensions, all scores are given as percents. The *Program Effort Score* used below is the percent attained out of the 120 maximum for all 30 scores. Detailed results appear in Mauldin and Ross (1991).

1. **Repeated assessments show that most developing countries have improved their program efforts substantially since 1972.**

   1.a. Program effort scores now average 42 percent, within a range of 0 to 87 percent of the maximum of 120. Assessments in 1972, 1982, and 1989 produced mean program effort scores of 20, 29, and 42, respectively, rising by 45 percent between 1982 and 1989.

   1.b. Over time the distribution of countries by the program effort score has shifted favorably (*Figure 1*), with a systematic movement of most countries toward higher scores. In each period additional countries established programs, thus moving upward from zero, and those already possessing programs strengthened them, raising their scores.

   1.c. Improvement has been quite general. The overall score rose for each of the four components, and did so within every geographic region, between 1982 and 1989 (*Table 2*).

   1.d. Nevertheless, as of 1989, half of all family planning programs still scored less than half of the maximum.

2. **All programs, including the stronger[1] ones, are selective in their efforts among the 30 scores.**

   2.a. In general most emphasis goes to basic policy positions, to essential infrastructure items, and to the availability of four of the six birth control methods shown (*Figure 2*).

3. **Stronger programs exceed weaker ones on every one of the 30 scores, but the differences are sharpest on outreach items.**

Table 1 Population concentration in the 20 largest developing countries

Largest developing countries	Population (000)	Percent of LDC total	Cumulative percent
1. China	1,139,060	27.9	27.9
2. India	853,094	20.9	48.8
3. Indonesia	184,283	4.5	53.3
4. Brazil	150,368	3.7	57.0
5. Pakistan	122,626	3.0	60.0
6. Bangladesh	115,593	2.8	62.8
7. Nigeria	108,542	2.7	65.5
8. Mexico	88,598	2.2	67.7
9. Vietnam	66,693	1.6	69.3
10. Philippines	62,413	1.5	70.8
11. Turkey	55,868	1.4	72.2
12. Thailand	55,702	1.4	73.6
13. Iran	54,607	1.3	74.9
14. Egypt	52,426	1.3	76.2
15. Ethiopia	49,240	1.2	77.4
16. North Korea	42,793	1.0	78.4
17. Myanmar	41,675	1.0	79.4
18. Zaire	35,568	.9	80.3
19. South Africa	35,282	.9	81.2
20. Colombia	32,978	.8	82.0
LDC total	4,085,640		

Note: LDC = less developed countries in United Nations statistical series.
Source: United Nations, 1991.

Program Effort

POLICY AND STAGE-SETTING ACTIVITIES

*1. Official government policy on fertility/family planning and population growth
*2. Favorable statements by government leaders
3. Level of family planning program leadership within government
4. Minimum legal age at marriage at least 18 for females; extent of enforcement
*5. Laws permitting contraceptive imports; in-country manufacture
6. Legalization of mass-media advertising of contraceptives
7. Involvement of numerous ministries and government agencies
*8. Percentage of total program budget from in-country sources

SERVICE AND SERVICE-RELATED ACTIVITIES

9. Involvement of private-sector agencies
10. Use of government personnel to carry out program; accountability at all levels
11. Community-based distribution (CBD)
12. Social marketing programs
*13. Postpartum family planning programs
*14. Home visiting by family planning workers
15. Adequate administrative structure and staff
*16. Adequate training programs
17. Extent that staff carry out assigned tasks
*18. Adequate logistics and transport
19. Adequate supervision
*20. Use of mass media
21. Incentives and/or disincentives

RECORD-KEEPING AND EVALUATION

*22. Collection, reporting, and feedback on clinic records
*23. Evaluation
24. Management use of evaluation findings to improve program

AVAILABILITY AND ACCESSIBILITY OF FERTILITY CONTROL METHODS

**25. Male sterilization
**26. Female sterilization
***27. Oral contraceptives (or injectables, if more popular)
***28. Condoms (or other barrier method, if more popular)
***29. IUDs
*30. Safe induced abortion

*Included in 1972 program effort scale
**Items 25-26 included as one item in 1972 program effort scale
***Included as two items in 1972 program effort scale

Figure 1 Distribution of program effort scores, 1972, 1982, and 1989

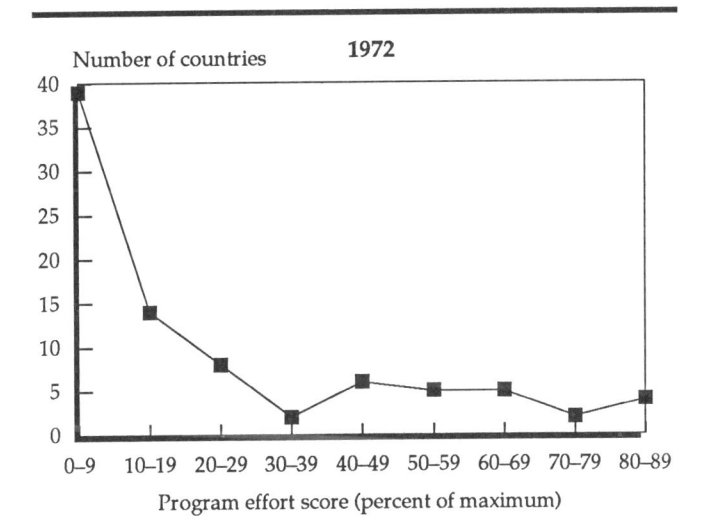

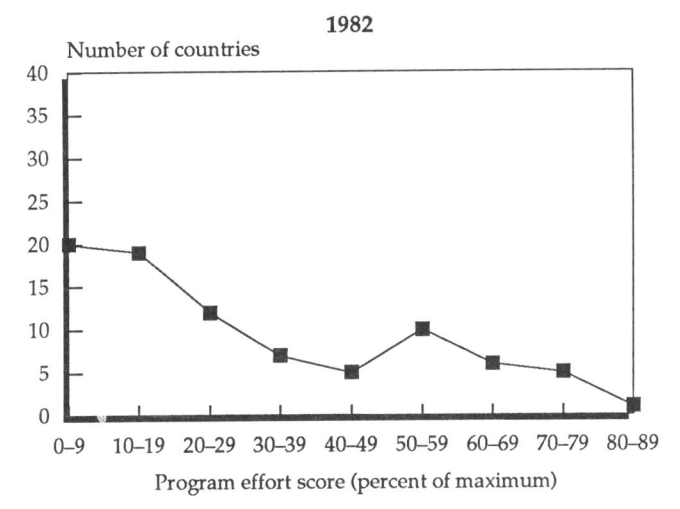

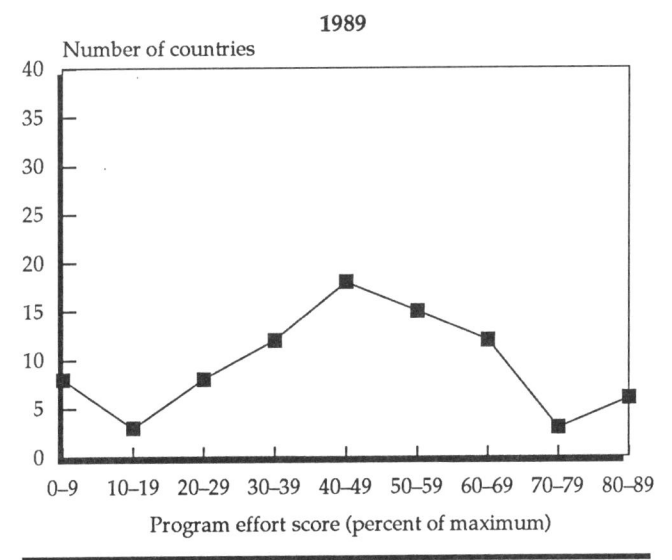

1972

1982

1989

Program effort score (percent of maximum)

Source: Population Council Databank, 1993.

Table 2 Family planning program effort scores (% of maximum), by component, according to region, 1982 and 1989

Component and year	All countries	East Asia	South Asia	Sub-Saharan Africa	Middle East/ North Africa	Latin America
Program effort						
1982	29	63	42	15	20	40
1989	44	64	52	36	33	54
Change	15	1	10	21	13	14
Policy and stage setting						
1982	34	66	45	25	26	39
1989	47	67	55	45	32	48
Change	13	1	10	20	6	9
Service and service related						
1982	25	58	38	12	16	34
1989	42	60	49	35	32	49
Change	17	2	11	23	16	15
Record keeping						
1982	29	57	43	13	21	42
1989	50	62	51	44	39	62
Change	21	5	8	31	18	20
Availability						
1982	31	76	45	10	21	53
1989	44	71	56	26	32	68
Change	13	−5	11	16	11	15

Note: The percentages are calculated by unit weights, not population weights.
Source: Mauldin and Ross, 1991.

3.a. The outreach items that differentiate best between stronger and weaker programs are community-based distribution of contraceptives, social marketing of contraceptives at subsidized prices, postpartum programs, and home visiting

4. **Weaker programs that improve over time do so selectively, rising on certain scores more than others.**

    4.a. Between 1982 and 1989, 19 programs moved from the weaker to the stronger group. Termed "shift countries," these improved on nearly all 30 scores, but especially on the three infrastructure items of task completion, administrative structure, and training, as well as on the use of mass media, on the management use of evaluation resources, and on making female sterilization more widely available.

5. **Some programs are constricted by formal barriers.**

    5.a. Controls on contraceptive imports, legal prohibitions against certain methods, and bans on the use of mass media all exist in some countries. In addition, medical barriers exist that involve elaborate screening procedures, multiple visits for examinations, and other impediments to contraceptive adoption (Shelton et al., 1992; Ross et al., 1992).

6. **Most contraceptive use in the developing world is program supplied, though regional variation exists** (*Table 3*). (See Chapter 1, for details on the method mix.)

Figure 2 Program effort scores, 1989, stronger vs. weaker programs

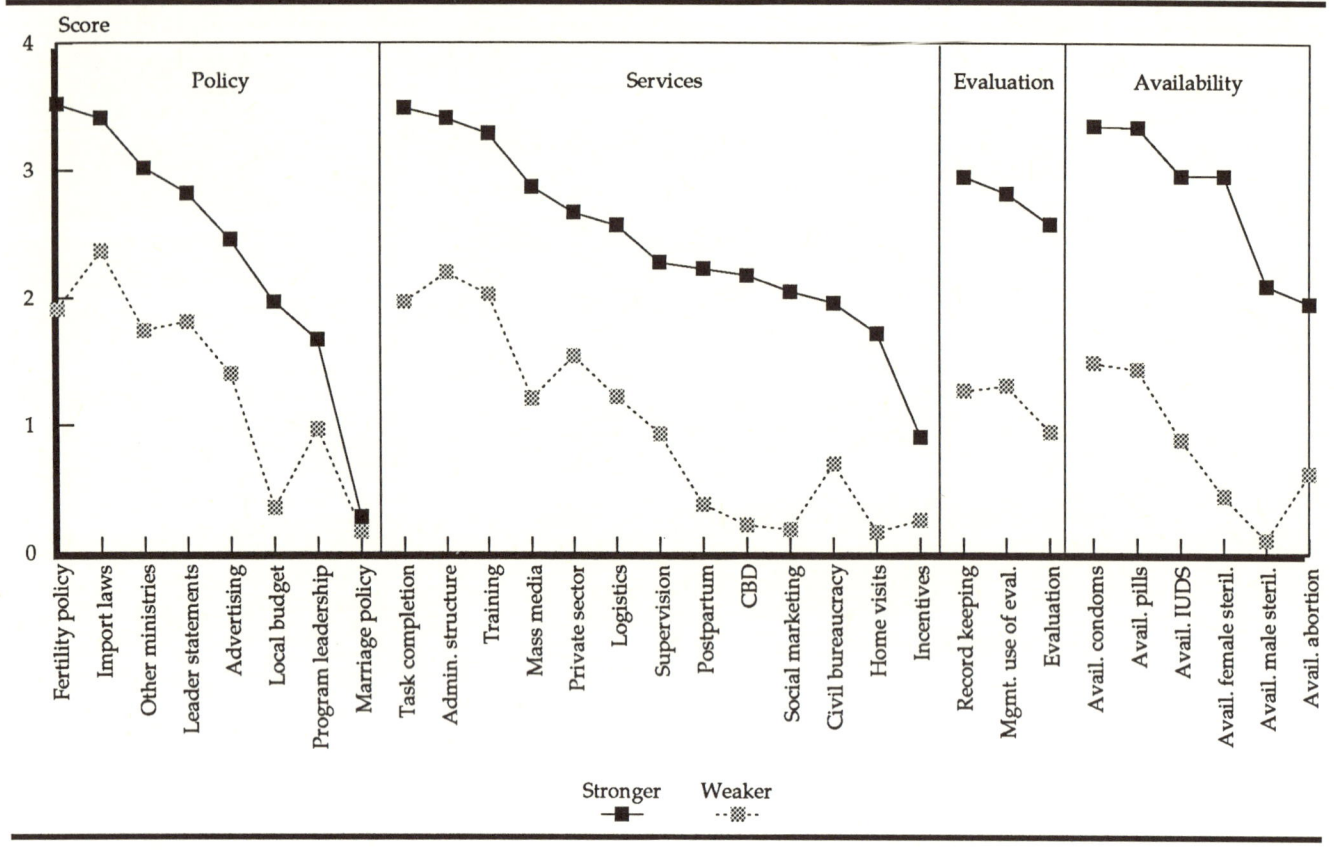

[Chart showing Score (0-4) across four categories: Policy, Services, Evaluation, Availability, comparing Stronger (solid line) vs Weaker (dashed line) programs]

Policy items: Fertility policy, Import laws, Other ministries, Leader statements, Advertising, Local budget, Program leadership, Marriage policy

Services items: Task completion, Admin. structure, Training, Mass media, Private sector, Logistics, Supervision, Postpartum, CBD, Social marketing, Civil bureaucracy, Home visits, Incentives

Evaluation items: Record keeping, Mgmt. use of eval., Evaluation

Availability items: Avail. condoms, Avail. pills, Avail. IUDS, Avail. female steril., Avail. male steril., Avail. abortion

Stronger ■— Weaker ··※··

Source: Population Council Databank, 1993.

6.a. Over 80 percent of all contraceptive users receive their supplies and services from public-sector programs. Essentially all of this use is of the modern methods (sterilization, IUD, pill, injectable, and condom).

6.b. Regional variation in the source of supply, however, is considerable (*Figure 3*). The proportions in *Table 3* vary from 99 percent publicly supplied for East Asia (heavily China) down to 29 percent publicly supplied for North Africa and the Middle East. The figure for Latin America is also low, at 38 percent; however, the "private sector" there includes many non-profit organizations, such as the Profamilia program in Colombia, which provide a substantial share of contraceptive services.

7. There is no apparent trend for the private sector to supplant the public sector as a source of supply; nevertheless, the private sector is important in some countries.

7.a. Repeat surveys in 16 countries show the public sector gaining ground in eight countries and losing it in five, with no change in three (shift defined by a change of five percentage points between sectors) (Mauldin et al., 1993).

7.b. There is no apparent trend toward a larger role for the private sector in distributing resupply methods (the pill and condom). In 17 countries with national surveys that permit a division of source of supply by government, NGO, and commercial, time-trend patterns are obscure in some cases, with the remainder of countries equally balanced between shifts up and down for the private sector (Population Council Databank, 1993).

7.c. Cross et al. (1991) examined survey evidence in 13 countries to determine whether the private sector's share of supplies and services for modern contraceptive use increased during the 1980s (3–9 years between surveys). Contrary to expectations the private sector's share increased in only one country, declined in seven, and is holding steady in the rest. The pattern was essentially similar for the urban sector. Also, in 12 of the 13 countries, pharmacies clearly lost market share. Data from 27 surveys carried out in the 1980s (including the 13 countries above) showed the private sector's share of resupply meth-

Table 3 Percentage of contraceptive users relying upon the public sector, by region* and selected countries

Region and country	Number of users 1990 (000)	Number of users in public sector (000)	Public sector users as percent of all users
East Asia			
China	167,722	167,722	100.0
South Korea	5,821	4,977	85.5
Entire region	177,117	175,218	98.9
South Asia			
India	75,338	57,068	75.8
Indonesia	17,249	13,074	75.8
Bangladesh	7,262	5,526	76.1
Thailand	6,763	5,539	81.9
Vietnam	5,655	5,457	96.5
Entire region	119,340	91,211	76.4
Middle East/ North Africa			
Turkey	6,547	1,243	19.0
Egypt	3,666	846	23.1
Morocco	1,392	868	62.4
Tunisia	635	485	76.4
Entire region	12,609	3,651	29.0
Sub-Saharan Africa			
Nigeria	1,315	487	37.1
Kenya	1,224	599	49.0
Zimbabwe	777	703	90.5
Ghana	437	133	30.6
Botswana	91	86	94.2
Entire region	5,870	3,144	53.6
Latin America			
Brazil	18,446	4,998	27.1
Mexico	8,507	5,257	61.8
Colombia	3,680	835	22.7
Peru	1,802	883	49.0
Ecuador	825	265	32.2
Dominican Republic	616	271	44.0
Entire region	35,948	13,533	37.6
Total	350,884	286,757	81.7

*Regional totals are only for countries with known numbers of total contraceptive users and users in the public sector. These countries include 92 percent of all users in the developing world.
Source: Population Council Databank, estimates based on national surveys.

Figure 3 Source of supply for contraceptive users in three developing regions (available data)

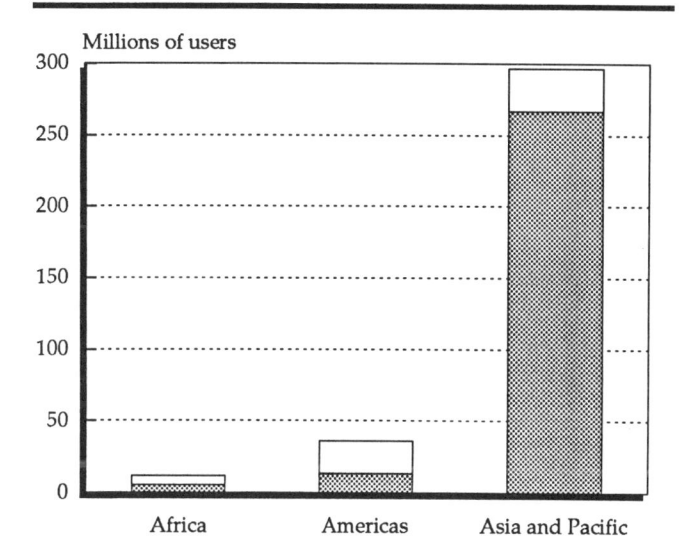

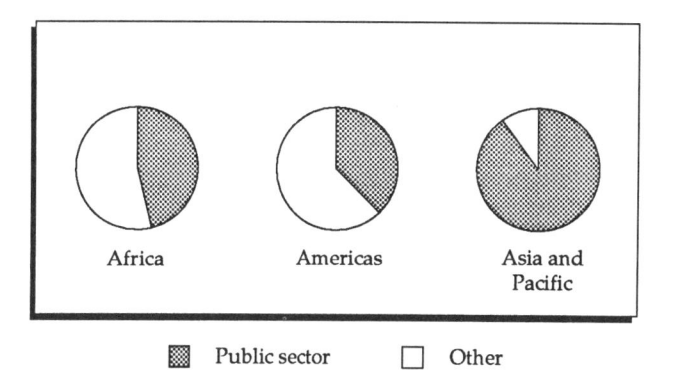

Source: Population Council Databank, 1993.

ods to be greater than that of long-acting methods, but time trends were not part of that analysis.

8. **The overall prevalence of contraceptive use is related to the number of methods made available.**

   8.a. Adding a new contraceptive method to those available in an existing program increases prevalence by about 12 percentage points and decreases the crude birth rate by 5.3 points. The effect of availability does not diminish when other elements of family planning program strength are taken into account (Jain, 1989).[2]

   8.b. The introduction of major new contraceptive methods has resulted in jumps in contraceptive prevalence; programs have sometimes fostered such introduction on a large scale (Freedman and Freedman, 1992).

   8.c. Programs that offer a number of methods increase the likelihood that users will find a method appropriate to their needs, leading to higher prevalence levels. Although other factors affect the relationship, the association is clearly suggestive of benefits that follow broadened method availability.[3]

Number of methods available	Contraceptive prevalence (%)
0	9
1–2	25
3–4	42
5–6	64

   8.d. In Matlab, Bangladesh, contraceptive prevalence rose from 7 percent to 20 percent when injectables were provided at the household level. The introduction of sterilization services was accompanied by another 10 percentage point increase in prevalence. A household visitation program to insert IUDs increased prevalence yet again. Although the new methods were associated with excellent continuation rates, they were not the only elements that contributed to increased prevalence, since other program improvements occurred simultaneously (Phillips et al., 1988, 1989).

8.e. In an experiment in Kaoshiung City, Taiwan, pills were added to the method mix to test the effect on IUD acceptance. Subsequently, IUD acceptance continued to rise, and there was a net increase in total program acceptors. The pill was then added to the island-wide program (Cernada and Lu, 1972).

8.f. The addition of the pill to large-scale programs in Thailand, Taiwan, South Korea, and Hong Kong, and the addition of the condom in India, produced net increases in contraceptive prevalence (Freedman and Berelson, 1976). After the Nirodh condom was added to the private sector in India, with accompanying publicity, condom sales rose from about 600,000 per month to about 7,000,000, of which 80 percent were the Nirodh type (Jain, 1973).

8.g. Method-specific failure rates (see Chapter 7) are lower in countries with high family planning effort scores (Moreno and Goldman, 1990, evidence from 15 DHS surveys). By offering a wider choice of methods, including low-failure methods, strong programs may help direct users to methods best suited for them, and they may provide better counselling about how to use methods effectively; all of these efforts encourage higher prevalence levels.

8.h. Improved availability of contraceptive methods tends to raise contraceptive prevalence (Tsui and Ochoa, 1992, reviewing the body of post-1992 evidence). However, countries vary greatly in the variety of contraceptive methods they make available.

A method is defined as "available" if at least half of the population has ready access to it. The table below distributes the 65 countries with information according to the number of methods available:[4]

Number of methods available	Number of developing countries
0	21
1	6
2	6
3	10
4	5
5	8
6	7
7	2
	65

Thus, 21 countries fail to make *any* contraceptive method readily available to at least half the population. These countries, largely in Africa and the Middle East, represent one-third of the 65 with data.

8.i. The availability of methods in many parts of the developing world is restricted by sheer lack of outlets. Early programs addressed this problem by authorizing paramedics to provide pills and insert IUDs. The safety of IUD insertion by paraprofessionals is one of the strongest findings in the operations research literature (Foreit, 1991). In a Thailand experiment, auxiliary nurse-midwives in four provinces were trained to prescribe the pill with a checklist of contraindications, omitting pelvic examinations. The number of program acceptors rose over three-fold in a six month period, with no increase in the complication rate and with continuation as good as that among the clients of physicians. The new system was extended to all of Thailand, raising the number of pill outlets from 350 to about 4,000 (Rosenfield and Limcharoen, 1972, cited in Foreit, 1991).

8.j. Outlets have been increased through other means, such as community-based distribution (see Chapter 3), contraceptive social marketing (see Chapter 4), postpartum programs (see Chapter 5), and mobile teams; there are also outlets at military and some workplace sites and schools.

9. **Programs that encourage adoption of long-acting methods among couples who wish to substantially delay or permanently prevent births can decrease the risk of contraceptive failure, the costs of distributing resupply methods, and the burden of recruiting new users to replace dropouts.**

9.a. To *maintain* a contraceptive prevalence level of approximately 75 percent (when the annual discontinuation rate is 60 percent, as it is with some methods in some countries), programs must recruit 45 acceptors annually for every 100 MWRA. Only 15 acceptors per 100 married women are needed when the annual discontinuation rate is 20 percent. To *increase* prevalence when discontinuation is high, the numbers of acceptors required are even greater than those needed to maintain it (Jain, 1989).

9.b. Even when discontinuation is low, prevalence will decline unless new users appear each year to replace dropouts and to keep up with the growth in the number of eligible couples. For the developing world as a whole, 100 million new users will be needed during the 1990–2000 decade just to keep prevalence at its 1990 level of 51 percent. To raise prevalence to 59 percent by 2000, consistent with the United Nations medium population projection, will require an additional 86 million users (Mauldin and Ross, 1992).

10. **The influence of contraceptive effectiveness on fertility depends upon the level of prevalence.**

   10.a. When prevalence is low, that is, when few people use a method, contraceptive effectiveness has little impact on the birth rate. For example, when prevalence is 30 percent, an increase in overall method effectiveness from 50 percent to 90 percent will lower the birth rate only modestly. But when prevalence is high, the change in effectiveness applies to most of the population, and the impact on the birth rate can be large.

11. **Contraceptive use is closely associated with program effort, regardless of socioeconomic setting.**

   11.a. Within each socioeconomic setting, the level of contraceptive use rises as program effort improves (*Figure 4*; countries weighted equally). Successive analyses for different time periods have found these patterns to be consistent (Freedman and Berelson, 1976; Mauldin and Berelson, 1978; Lapham and Mauldin, 1984, 1985; Mauldin and Ross, 1991).

   11.b. Cross-country analyses that take account of both individual and country sources of variation suggest that program effort raises contraceptive prevalence (Freedman and Freedman, 1992).

12. **Fertility levels are also closely associated with program effort.**

   12.a. Again, within each socioeconomic setting, fertility is generally lower where program effort is greater (*Table 4*). Analyses for successive time periods have found consistent patterns (sources as in 11.a. above).

   12.b. One study, based upon regression methods, relates the decline in TFR to the effects of program effort and of socioeconomic development (as measured by the UN Human Development Index). The average net program effect, weighted across 48 countries, has been to reduce the TFR by 1.4 births per woman. This implies that organized programs (both government and NGO) "...have been responsible for fully half of the fertility decline from 6.4 to 3.9 births per woman between the pretransition period and the late 1980s" (Bongaarts, 1993). The results are consistent with those obtained in an earlier study (Bongaarts et al., 1990).

   12.c. Major fertility declines have occurred in the presence of strong family planning programs where social and economic conditions were believed to be unfavorable; prominent examples are China, Indonesia, and Thailand (Freedman and Freedman, 1992). Additional examples include Bangladesh and certain states of India.

   12.d. Reviews of earlier evidence also support the conclusion that organized family planning programs can affect the course of fertility (Hermalin, 1982; Forrest and Ross, 1978).

   12.e. Areal variations in contraceptive prevalence and fertility within a single country are associated with variations in the strength and quality of program effort, as in Indonesia, Malaysia, and Taiwan (Freedman and Freedman, 1992).

13. **Program effort is only partly determined by the social and economic setting. It is not simply a reflection of a country's level of development.**

   13.a. Among countries that rank high on social setting, program effort in 1989 varied: weak or very weak/none in seven countries, moderate in 10, and strong in only five. Overall correlations between program effort and social setting varied from 0.14 to 0.67, depending upon the measures used (Mauldin and Ross, 1991).

   13.b. Nevertheless, it is difficult to develop a strong program in a poor social setting, with its fragile infrastructures of transportation, communication, and trained personnel. In the 1989 study only one country, Bangladesh, ranked low on social setting and high on program effort, and only two countries, In-

Figure 4 Relation of contraceptive prevalence to program effort, by socioeconomic setting

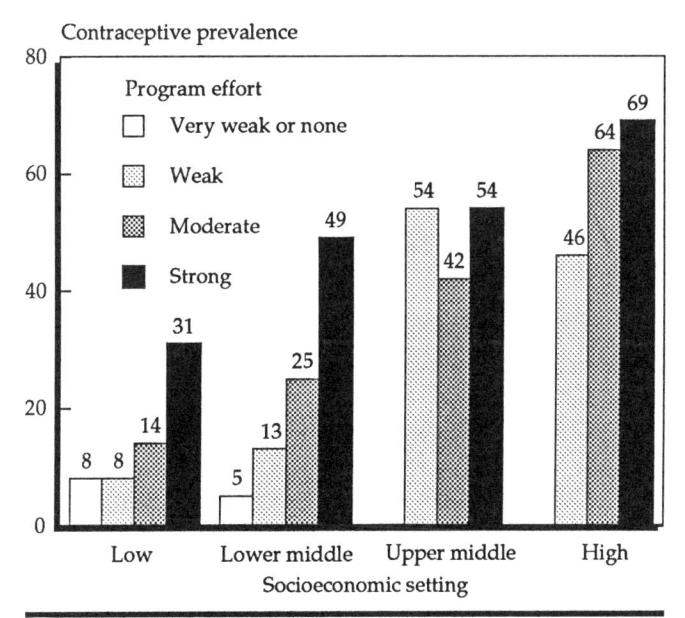

Source: Population Council Databank

Table 4 Relation of total fertility rate (1990) to program effort (1989) and social setting (1985)

Social setting	Program effort: Strong		Medium		Weak		Very weak/none		Mean
High	1. Mexico	3.34†	1. Venezuela	3.62	1. Jordan	5.84	1. Iraq	6.15	
	2. Mauritius	1.95	2. Lebanon	3.59	2. Brazil	3.31	2. U.A.E.	4.56	
	3. Taiwan	1.70	3. Costa Rica	3.14	3. Argentina	2.87	3. Kuwait	3.65	
	4. South Korea	1.69	4. Colombia	3.03	4. Uruguay	2.38	Sub-total	4.79	
	Sub-total	2.17	5. Panama	3.01	Sub-total	3.60			3.09
			6. Trin. & Tobago	2.83					
			7. Chile	2.69					
			8. Jamaica	2.52					
			9. North Korea	2.45					
			10. Cuba	1.85					
			11. Singapore	1.80					
			Sub-total	2.77					
Upper-middle	1. Botswana	5.00	1. Guatemala	5.57	1. Syria	6.51	1. Saudi Arabia	7.12	
	2. El Salvador	4.68	2. Zimbabwe	5.56	2. Congo	6.29	2. Libya	6.76	
	3. Tunisia	3.74	3. Iran	4.96	3. Algeria	5.14	Sub-total	6.94	
	4. Indonesia	3.29	4. S. Africa	4.32	4. Paraguay	4.46			4.41
	5. Sri Lanka	2.57	5. Egypt	4.26	5. Turkey	3.49			
	6. Thailand	2.40	6. Philippines	4.12	Sub-total	5.18			
	7. China	2.35	7. Ecuador	4.08					
	Sub-total	3.43	8. Peru	3.79					
			9. Malaysia	3.75					
			10. Dom. Republic	3.55					
			11. Guyana	2.58					
			Sub-total	4.23					
Lower-middle	1. India	4.20	1. Zambia	7.20	1. Yemen	7.49	1. Ivory Coast	7.41	
	2. Vietnam	3.90	2. Kenya	6.70	2. Tanzania	7.11	2. Oman	7.12	
	Sub-total	4.05	3. Ghana	6.34	3. Cameroon	6.90	3. Liberia	6.75	
			4. Pakistan	6.22	4. Nigeria	6.75	4. Laos	6.69	5.95
			5. Honduras	5.24	5. Madagascar	6.55	5. Namibia	5.92	
			6. Morocco	4.51	6. Cen. Afr. Rep.	6.19	6. Gabon	5.17	
			Sub-total	6.04	7. Zaire	6.09	7. Cambodia	4.56	
					8. Bolivia	5.93	8. Myanmar	3.86	
					9. Lesotho	5.78	Sub-total	5.93	
					10. Papua N.G.	5.05			
					11. Haiti	4.89			
					Sub-total	6.25			
Low	1. Bangladesh	5.33	1. Nepal	5.74	1. Rwanda	8.14	1. Malawi	7.60	
	Sub-total	5.33	Sub-total	5.74	2. Uganda	7.30	2. Somalia	6.60	
					3. Benin	7.11	3. Mauritania	6.50	
					4. Mali	7.11	4. Sudan	6.36	
					5. Niger	7.11	5. Chad	5.84	
					6. Guinea	7.00	Sub-total	6.58	
					7. Afghanistan	6.85			
					8. Burundi	6.79			
					9. Ethiopia	6.78			6.58
					10. Togo	6.58			
					11. Sierra Leone	6.50			
					12. Burkina Faso	6.50			
					13. Angola	6.36			
					14. Guinea	6.33			
					15. Mozambique	6.31			
					16. Guinea-Bissau	5.78			
					17. Bhutan	5.53			
					Sub-total	6.71			
Mean		3.30		4.10		6.03		6.03	5.07

(Unit weights for means)
Note: Total fertility rate taken from 1990 United Nations medium estimate.
†Read: The total fertility rate is 3.34 in Mexico, which has a strong program effort and a high social setting.
Source: Population Council Databank, based on Mauldin and Ross, 1991.

dia and Vietnam, ranked in the lower middle social setting group and in the strong program effort group.

14. Socioeconomic differentials in contraceptive use tend to weaken under strong programs.

14.a. The adoption of birth control by disadvantaged sectors of the population in countries with strong programs has been very substantial, as in Taiwan and Indonesia, probably improving the equity and speed of fertility decline.

NOTES

1. "Stronger" programs are all those that rate higher than 45 on the program effort score; these include the "strong" and the "moderate" ones in Table 3. "Weaker" programs are all those at or below the 45 cutoff; these include the "weak" and "very weak/none" ones in Table 3.
2. Jain used data from Lapham and Mauldin (1984,1985) on family planning program strength from 100 developing countries in a regression model that predicted prevalence and birth rate as a function of a country's score on method availability.
3. Source: Population Council Databank.
4. As judged by observers in each country, reported in Ross et al. (1992), Table 14.

REFERENCES

Bongaarts, J. 1993. "The Fertility Impact of Family Planning Programs." The Population Council, *Research Division Working Papers*, No. 47.

Bongaarts, J., W.P. Mauldin, and J. Phillips. 1990. "The demographic impact of family planning programs." *Studies in Family Planning* 21(6):299–310.

Cernada, G. and L. Lu. 1972. "The Kaoshiung study." *Studies in Family Planning* 3(8):198–203.

Cross, E.H., V.H. Poole, R.E. Levine, and R.M. Cornelius. 1991. "Contraceptive Source and the For-Profit Private Sector in Third World Family Planning: Evidence and Implications From Trends in Private Sector Use in the 1980s." Paper presented at the Population Association Annual Meeting, March.

Foreit, J. 1991. "Reaching more users: More methods, more outlets, more promotion." *Operations Research: Helping Family Planning Programs Work Better*, Progress in Clinical and Biological Research. 371:215–231.

Forrest, J.D. and J.A. Ross. 1978. "Fertility effects of family planning programs: A methodological review." *Social Biology* 25:145–163.

Freedman, R. and B. Berelson. 1976. "The record of family planning programs." *Studies in Family Planning* 7(1):1–40.

Freedman, R. and D. Freedman. 1992. "The role of family planning programmes as a fertility determinant." In *Family Planning Programmes and Fertility*. J.F. Phillips and J.A. Ross, eds. Oxford: Oxford University Press.

Hermalin, A. 1982. "Issues in the comparative analysis of techniques for evaluating family planning programmes." *Evaluation of the Impact of Family Planning Programmes on Fertility: Sources of Variance*. Population Studies No. 76. ST/ESA/SER.A/76. New York: United Nations Department of International Economic and Social Affairs, pp. 29–40.

Jain, A.K. 1989. "Fertility reduction and the quality of family planning services." *Studies in Family Planning* 20(1):1–16.

Lapham, R.J., and W.P. Mauldin. 1984. "Family planning program effort and birthrate decline in developing countries." *International Family Planning Perspectives* 10(4):109–118.

Lapham R.J., and W.P. Mauldin. 1985. "Contraceptive prevalence: The influence of organized family planning programs." *Studies in Family Planning* 16(3):117–137.

Mauldin, W.P. and B. Berelson. 1978. "Conditions of fertility decline in developing countries, 1965–75," *Studies in Family Planning*, 9(5):89–148.

Mauldin, W.P., and J.A. Ross. 1991. "Family planning programs: Efforts and results, 1982–89." *Studies in Family Planning* 22(6): 350–367.

Mauldin, W.P. and S.J. Segal. 1993. "IUD use throughout the world: Past, present and future." In *A New Look at IUDs* C.W. Bardin and D.R. Mishell, eds. Stoneham, MA: Butterworth.

Mauldin, W.P., S.J. Segal, and S. Sinding. 1993. *Prevalence of Contraceptive Use: A Chart Book*. Forthcoming. Page 32.

Moreno, L. and N. Goldman. 1990. "Contraceptive failure rates in developing countries: Evidence from the Demographic and Health Surveys." Unpublished.

Phillips, J.F., R. Simmons, M.A. Koenig, and J. Chakraborty. 1988. "Determinants of reproductive change in a traditional society: Evidence for Matlab, Bangladesh." *Studies in Family Planning* 19(6):313–334.

Phillips, J.F., M.B. Hossain, A.A.Z. Huque, and J. Akbar. 1989. "A case study of contraceptive introduction: Domiciliary depot-medroxy progesterone acetate services in Rural Bangladesh." Chapter in *Demographic and Programmatic Consequences of Contraceptive Innovations*. Eds. S. Segal, A.O. Tsui, and S.M. Rogers. New York: Plenum Press, pp. 227–248.

Rosenfield, A. and C. Limcharoen. 1972. "Auxiliary midwife prescription of oral contraceptives." *American Journal of Obstetrics and Gynecology* 114:942–49.

Ross, J.A., W.P. Mauldin, S.R. Green, and E.R. Cooke. 1992. *Family Planning and Child Survival Programs as Assessed in 1991*. New York: The Population Council.

Shelton, J.D., M.A. Angle, and R.A. Jacobstein. 1992. "Medical barriers to access to family planning." *The Lancet* 340:1334–1335

Tsui, A.O. and L.H. Ochoa. 1992. "Service proximity as a determinant of contraceptive behaviour: Evidence from cross-national studies of survey data." In *Family Planning Programmes and Fertility*. Eds. J.F. Phillips and J.A. Ross. Oxford University Press.

United Nations. 1991. *World Population Prospects 1990*. Department of International Economics and Social Affairs. Population Studies No. 120 (ST/ESA/SER.A.120). New York: United Nations.

Chapter 3

COMMUNITY-BASED DISTRIBUTION

The essential feature of community-based distribution (CBD) programs is that they deliver services and information to populations beyond the reach of fixed clinics and health centers. They cover villages and sometimes urban slums where services are scarce. Usually, CBD projects use lay workers, often unpaid, to distribute supplies from small depots or to deliver them door to door. They were established on the premise that without them, large populations would have limited access to services and would continue to have a low prevalence of contraceptive use. (For general reviews of CBD programs for family planning and related health objectives see Foreit et al. [1978]; Gallen and Rinehart [1986]; Kols and Wawer [1982]; and Osborn and Reinke [1981]).

COVERAGE

1. In numerous countries, substantial proportions of the rural population are reported to be covered by CBD programs, according to country informants (estimates subject to informant perceptions) (Ross et al., 1992, Table 12).

    1.a. By region, the proportions covered are as follows:

    *   Latin America: 30–40 percent in the Dominican Republic, Ecuador, El Salvador, and Guatemala; 60 percent in Mexico; 70 percent in Honduras; and "most of the rural and urban population" in Colombia.

    *   Middle East/North Africa: 22 percent in Syria; 60 percent in Morocco.

    *   Asia: 70 percent rural and 35 percent urban in Indonesia; 80 percent rural and 90 percent urban in Thailand; 90 percent in South Korea; 90 percent rural and 95 percent urban in China; "most of the rural and urban population" in Bangladesh and Taiwan.

    *   Sub-Saharan Africa: 13 percent in Botswana; 30 percent in both Kenya and Zimbabwe; and "most of the population, both rural and urban" in Mauritius. Zimbabwe has an exceptional program. In the 1984 national survey, one out of every five women in union reported a visit by a CBD worker, most within the last month. Among rural women currently using a modern contraceptive, 42 percent obtained it from the distributors, and among those not using a modern method, 35 percent knew of the CBD program as a potential source; about half of these women had used the CBD system in the past. About one in five nonusers reported visits by CBD distributors, about half within the last month (Zinanga, 1990).

PROVIDERS

2. The number of providers in CBD programs ranges from few to many, and the level of activity varies among workers, especially where they are unpaid (Ross et al., 1992).

    2.a. The range of the numbers of providers in CBD programs is:

    *   1,000 to 4,000 workers in several countries: Honduras, Kenya, Brazil's BEMFAM program (private family planning association), Guatemala, Taiwan, Ecuador, Syria, and South Korea.

    *   7,500 providers in Morocco; 11,000 in Turkey; and about 12,000 in Mexico (Ministry of Health system).

    *   19,000 providers in Indonesia (covering a reported 67,000 villages and hamlets); 28,000 in Bangladesh; and 970,000 reported for China (covering 800,000 villages) (Ross et al., 1992, Table 12).

EFFORT LEVELS

3. Countries can be distributed according to the extent of effort they give to their CBD programs, using a scale from 0 to 4. This scale is based upon the proportion of the total population that is covered by the CBD program.

    3.a. Many programs operate only in the rural sector, which dilutes the score; however, the score also reflects urban programs where they exist.

Score	1982	1989
0–.99	74	69
1.0–1.99	10	6
2.0–2.99	11	7
3.0–3.99	2	5
4.0[a]	6	16
No. of countries	103	103

Source: Population Council Databank, 1992
[a] 4.0 is used for all values of 4.0 and above.

3.b. Most countries fall low on the scale, because they have not yet established a CBD program or because its coverage is still restricted to only part of the country. Sixteen countries fall at high values; the rest are spread thinly at intermediate points.

3.c. Between 1982 and 1989, the distribution of scores shifted favorably, with 21 countries instead of eight at scores of three or above.

OUTCOMES

4. **Periodic reviews of CBD projects and programs have confirmed their positive effects upon contraceptive prevalence.**

4.a. "It has been postulated that substantial unmet demand exists for effective methods of fertility control and that community-based contraceptive distribution (CBD) systems can make significant inroads in meeting this demand at reasonable cost. Experience to date clearly confirms the validity of the thesis. Contraceptive prevalence rates have typically doubled from 15 percent or less to roughly 30 percent within a year or two after CBD program initiation. The question is no longer the feasibility of the CBD approach; rather, the issue is how the approach can be applied most effectively and efficiently" (Osborn and Reinke, 1981, reviewing 28 CBD projects).

4.b. "Operations research projects around the world have demonstrated that providing services through home visits and/or local supply depots can significantly increase contraceptive use. While some studies are more rigorous and conclusive than others, all of the studies in rural areas with initially low levels of use found increased use after community-based services became available" (Gallen and Rinehart, 1986).

4.c. "Operations research studies have already shown that CBD can be an extremely effective approach for supplementing clinic services, especially in rural areas. For family planning, they have also shown significant and rapid increases in contraceptive usage in rural areas" (Kennedy, 1986).

4.d. CBD "... is less costly than clinic services, easier for many people to reach, and available in a broad range of settings. Family planning services have been delivered by CBD for over 20 years; by the mid 80s CBD services were available in over 40 countries, largely in Asia and Latin America, but increasingly in Africa" (WHO, 1989).

4.e. Early CBD experience for acceptance, continuation, and prevalence produced the following outcomes (Foreit et al., 1978):

* Acceptance: In nine CBD programs, acceptance rates for contraception ranged from 10–16 percent of couples in three cases, 29–49 percent in four, and 69 percent in two.

* Continuation: Twelve-month continuation rates in six CBD programs for the pill were 33–41 percent in four programs and 56–76 percent in two other programs. For condoms, rates were 42 percent, 57 percent, and 82 percent in three programs.

* Prevalence: Prevalence of contraceptive use rose by 7–14 percentage points in four projects, to levels of 15 percent, 31 percent, 35 percent, and 38 percent, depending upon the project.

DISTRIBUTION STRATEGIES

Much CBD experience can be expressed as *who* provides *what* to *whom* and by what *means*.

5. *Who*: **Distributors have usually but not always been unsalaried residents who are selected and trained by regular program staff.**

5.a. Various approaches are used to establish and maintain distributor motivation: close supervision, enhanced social position in the community, payments to cover transportation expenses, provision of shoes and rain gear, and so on. Some programs that charge clients for supplies permit the workers to keep part of that income (Bouzidi and Korte, 1990).

5.b. In Zimbabwe, the distributors are full-time, salaried workers on the regular government payroll, with full benefits. Distributors in Morocco are also full-time and salaried.

5.c. In Kenya, some 23 agencies provide village-based services, covering about 35 percent of rural administrative units; workers are generally volunteers, working under various compensation arrangements (Phillips and Lewis, 1992).

5.d. In Sudan, resident village midwives who had previously received nine months' formal training for midwifery were used as unpaid volunteers to distribute, door to door, oral rehydration solution (ORS) and contraceptive pills, and to provide nutrition education (El Tom et al., 1984, 1989; Lauro, 1987).

5.e. Both men and women have been used as distributors; in two Peruvian projects, male and female distributors were recruited, trained, and supervised through similar procedures. Males were found to distribute more condoms and females, more pills; overall, males did as well or better than females in total numbers of clients recruited and total couple-years of protection provided. By adding male distributors to the program to recruit more male clients, total prevalence may rise due to the increased availability of male methods, especially the condom (Foreit et al., 1992). In a Zaire project men and women performed about equally well as distributors; women were slightly more productive, as measured by couple-years of protection provided (Bertrand et al., 1989); (see also Townsend, 1991).

5.f. In general, paid workers recruited in sufficient numbers to cover a large population create a heavy cost burden, while unpaid workers often lack motivation. Consequently, some CBD programs have been difficult to maintain. Townsend's (1991) review stresses that "high turnover, together with the recurrent costs of recruitment and training, continues to be a characteristic of many programs using volunteer community workers."

6. *What*: **The usual commodities given for family planning are pills and condoms, sometimes spermicides, and (rarely) injectables.**

    6.a. Other services include the delivery of oral rehydration supplies, malaria tablets, iron supplements, and anti-parasite preparations.

    6.b. Distributors also refer clients to health facilities for the clinical methods of IUDs, injectables, and sterilization, as well as immunization and other MCH services.

    6.c. Among 31 countries replying to a 1987 questionnaire, 16 reported that their CBD programs provided family planning and MCH services, as well as immunization referral. Nine provided family planning services only; three offered family planning and immunization referral; and three provided only MCH or immunization referral. Thus, 28 of the 31 provided some type of family planning service (Ross et al., 1988).

7. *To Whom*: **Most CBD programs are directed at rural populations. Some, such as the one in Morocco and a pilot project in Zaire, have included urban components.**

    7.a. The Zimbabwe CBD program selected rural areas of a fixed size (radius about 15 km), to control the worker's travel time. Relatively underserved areas were chosen, each one fairly close to a health center or clinic, which could handle referrals and treatment of side effects. All households containing eligible women are visited regularly for recruitment and resupply purposes (Zinanga, 1990).

8. *By What Means*: **Workers have operated in three modes: (a) by maintaining a small depot of supplies to which local residents come, (b) by going door to door, and (c) by holding educational meetings (in schools, in health facilities, and elsewhere in the community).**

    8.a. Combinations are employed: An initial home visit may be followed by one or two reinforcement visits during which supplies are given, after which the recipient must go to a depot or other facility for resupply. However, in some large programs, such as those in Bangladesh, Zimbabwe, and the Sudan, home visits continue on a permanent basis for resupply, referrals, and additional recruitment (rural locations only) (Gallen and Rinehart, 1986).

9. **CBD programs take different forms, even within the same country, depending partly upon each organization's character, its adaptations to local circumstances, and its general role in the society.**

    9.a. In Kenya, many voluntary associations maintain CBD programs, with a remarkable diversity in the way they go about their work. *Table 1* documents the variation that exists in the projects studied (Phillips and Lewis, 1992). All, however, reflect the common theme of carrying services out beyond the catchment areas of fixed clinics.

CHARGES FOR SERVICES

10. **Most countries charge for CBD services.**

    10.a. Among the 48 countries possessing a large CBD program in a 1991 survey, 31 charge for supplies and services and only seven do not (10 unknowns). However, charges are usually nominal or small (Ross et al., 1992, Table 12).

Table 1 CBD agencies, by type of implementation strategy, Kenya

CBD agency	Recruitment scheme	CBD agent	Financing	Client fee	IEC strategy	Political liason	Supervisory scheme	Outreach strategy
FPAK	Clinic with community participation	Paid staff	External	None	Household and clinic based	Weak	Strong, clinic based	Household canvassing
DFH/MOH	Clinic	Unpaid volunteers	Public sector	None	Clinic based	Weak	Weak	Not specified
MWYO	Community	Paid volunteers	Community plus external	None	Village economic group	Strong	Village coordination and technical support	Women's self help groups
CHAK	Church	Unpaid volunteers	Community plus external	Health service fees	Mobile teams and clinic based	Weak	Weak	Depots
CORAT	Church volunteers	Unpaid volunteers	Community	Health service	Mobile teams	Weak	Weak	Depots
PCEA	Clinic outreach	Paid	External fees only	Health service	Household	Weak	Strong	Household canvassing and depots
CMA	Clinic outreach	Paid	External	None	Clinic and household	Strong	Strong	Household canvassing

Notes: FPAK — Family Planning Association of Kenya; DFH/MOH — Division of Family Planning, Ministry of Health; MWYO — Maendeleyo ya Wanawake Organization; CHAK — Christian Health Association of Kenya; CORAT — Christian Organization Research Advisory Trust; PCEA — Presbyterian Church of East Africa (Chogoria); CMA — Crescent Medical Association.
Source: Phillips and Lewis, 1992, Table 2, p.17.

TRAINING

11. CBD workers are a distinct cadre in terms of their qualifications, work environment, and needs. They usually require specialized training, since they are not well educated or even literate, have little time to leave home for instruction courses, and must work most of the time without immediate supervision, unlike clinic personnel (Gallen and Rinehart, 1986).

11.a. Training usually takes from three days to two weeks, and trainers are usually regular program staff, or doctors and nurses on ad hoc assignments.

11.b. Phased training is usually needed wherever multiple duties are involved. In Sudan, it was found that training for a single function, with reinforcement in the field prior to training for the next function, was much more effective than simultaneous training for multiple functions (El Tom, 1985; El Tom et al., 1984, 1989).

11.c. Recurrent training for reinforcement of skills is needed for substantial proportions of workers. In the Guatemala APROFAM program, those CBD workers who were trained recently performed better than others on tests of contraceptive knowledge (Bertrand et al., 1981). In Ecuador, Ministry of Health community workers had low average scores on knowledge of course contents from their training one year previously (PRICOR, 1986).

12. **Individual training has been superior to group training in some trials.**

12.a. In Peru a traditional refresher course for CBD workers was compared with individual retraining that was conducted by each supervisor at the worker's own site. The latter resulted in 34 percent higher levels of family planning knowledge than did the group retraining. It also occupied much less of each distributor's time than attending the lengthy group course; moreover, nearly every distributor was contacted individually, whereas over one-third were absent from the group course (Leon, 1989).

12.b. Individual training also worked better in the Dominican Republic. There, a trial of "...one-on-one reinforcement of knowledge during supervision was 31 percent more effective ... than the traditional method of providing retraining to large groups of promoters. It also doubled the level of couple-months of protection achieved, while reducing by about 75 percent the percentage of pill users with contraindications" (Profamilia, 1990, cited in Townsend, 1991).

SUPERVISION

13. **Persistent, supportive supervision is essential to good worker performance.**

13.a. Reinforcement by supervisors of the basic knowledge of CBD distributors is important. In a Peruvian experiment distributors lacking regular reinforcement by supervisors lost about one-fifth of their family planning knowledge within five months of taking a basic course. Meanwhile, an experimental group to which supervisors gave systematic retraining improved their knowledge scores by 33 percent (Leon et al., 1990).

13.b. Studies from Bangladesh and Colombia found the following supervisor approaches to be associated with better worker performance: joint home visits with workers to observe their interaction with clients, questioning of clients about the worker's activities in the presence of the worker, discussion of clients' problems with the worker (Bernhart and Kamal, 1991; Gomez, 1981; both cited by Townsend, 1991).

13.c. The optimal frequency of supervisory visits is uncertain. Evidence from Guatemala, Turkey, Oyo State in Nigeria, and Ecuador supports frequent supervisory contacts. However, a change from monthly to quarterly supervisory visits in the Brazil BEMFAM program and in the Colombia Profamilia program did not appear to harm performance and saved time and money (Gallen and Rinehart, 1986).

REFERENCES

Bernhart, M.H. and G.M. Kamal. 1991. "Management of CBD programs in Bangladesh." Unpublished manuscript.

Bertrand, J.T. 1991. "Recent lessons from operations research on service delivery mechanisms." *Operations Research: Helping Family Planning Programs Work Better*. M. Seidman and M.C. Horn, eds. New York: Wiley-Liss Inc.

Bertrand, J.T., M.A. Pineda, R. Santiso, and S. De Monlina. 1981. "Evaluation of distributors' knowledge of contraceptives in the Guatemalan CBD program." Paper presented at the annual meeting of the Population Association of America, Washington, DC, 26–28 March.

Bouzidi, M. and R. Korte, eds. 1990. *Family Planning for Life: Experiences and Challenges for the 1990s*. London: International Planned Parenthood Federation.

El Tom, A.R. 1985. "The Sudan community-based health and family planning project: Description of a training course." In *Health and Family Planning in Community Based Distribution Programs*. M. Wawer, S. Huffman, D. Cebula, and R. Osborn, eds. Boulder, Colorado: Westview Press. Pp.417–422.

El Tom, A.R., N. Mubarak, S. Wesley, M.H. Matthews, and D. Lauro. 1984. "Developing the skills of illiterate health workers." *World Health Forum* 5(3):216–220.

El Tom, A.R., D. Lauro, A. Farah, R. McNamara, and E. Ali Ahmed. 1989. "Family planning in Sudan: A pilot project success story." *World Health Forum* 10(3/4):333–343.

Foreit, J. R., M. Gorosh, D. Gillespie, and C. G. Merritt. 1978. "Community-based and commercial contraceptive distribution: An inventory and appraisal." *Population Reports* Series J, No. 19, March.

Foreit, J. R., M. R. Garate, A. Brazzoduro, F. Guillen, M. Herrera, and F. C. Suarez. 1992. "A comparison of the performance of male and female CBD distributors in Peru." *Studies in Family Planning* 23(1)58–62.

Gallen, M. E. and W. Rinehart. 1986. "Operations research: Lessons for policy and programs." *Population Reports* Series J, No. 31.

Gomez, F. 1981. "Rural household delivery of contraceptives in Colombia." Bogota, Colombia: The Population Council (unpublished).

Kennedy, B. 1986. "Bringing family planning to the people in Sub-Saharan Africa." In *Proceedings of a Conference on Community-Based Distribution and Alternative Delivery Systems in Africa: Harare, Zimbabwe*. Washington, DC: American Public Health Association.

Kols, A.J. and M. J. Wawer. 1982. "Community-based health and family planning." *Population Reports* Series L–3, vol. 10 (6): L77–L111.

Lauro, D. 1987. "Sudan community-based family health project" *Proceedings of a Conference on Community-Based Distribution and Alternative Delivery Systems in Africa*, Harare, Zimbabwe. Washington, D.C.: American Public Health Association, p. 106–108.

Leon, F. 1989. "Comparación de conocimientos de distribuidores comunitarios en planificación familiar." Paper presented at the Second Latin American Congress on Family Planning, Rio de Janeiro, Brazil.

Leon, F. et al. 1990. "An experiment to improve the quality of care in a Peruvian community-based distribution program." Final Technical Report, Instituto Peruano de Paternidad Responsable (INPPARES) and The Population Council, Lima, Peru.

Mauldin, W.P. and R.J. Lapham. 1984. "Conditions of fertility decline in the LDCs: 1965–1980." Paper presented at the annual meeting of the Population Association of America, Minneapolis, Minnesota, 3–5 May.

Osborn, R. W. and W. A. Reinke, eds. 1981. *Community Based Distribution of Contraception: A Review of Field Experience*. Johns Hopkins Population Center, The Johns Hopkins University School of Hygiene and Public Health.

Phillips, J.F and G.L. Lewis. 1992. "Strategies for the community-based distribution of contraceptives in the Kenyan family planning program." Report prepared for the Population Council's Africa Operations Research and Technical Assistance Project, February (unpublished).

Primary Health Care Operations Research (PRICOR). 1986. "Training in Luna, Ecuador: Interim report." Unpublished manuscript.

Profamilia (Asociacion Dominicana Pro Bienestar de la Familia). 1990. "Strengthening human resources for CBD program expansion." Final Report to The Population Council.

Ross, J.A., M. Rich, J. Molzan, and M. Pensak. 1988. *Family Planning and Child Survival: 100 Developing Countries*. New York: Center for Population and Family Health, Columbia University.

Ross, J.A., W.P. Mauldin, S.R. Green, and E.R. Cooke. 1992. *Family Planning and Child Survival Programs as Assessed in 1991*. New York: The Population Council.

Townsend, J.W. 1991. "Effective family planning service components: Global lessons from operations research." In *Operations Research: Helping Family Planning Programs Work Better*. M. Seidman and M.C. Horn, eds. New York: Wiley-Liss Inc.

World Health Organization. 1989. *WHO Guidelines on Community-Based Distribution of Contraceptives in Family Planning Programmes*. (Unpublished manuscript).

Zinanga, A. 1990. "Community-based distribution programmes in Zimbabwe." In *Family Planning for Life: Experiences and Challenges for the 1990s*. M. Bouzidi and R. Korte, eds. London: International Planned Parenthood Federation (IPPF). Pp. 37–44.

Chapter 4

CONTRACEPTIVE SOCIAL MARKETING[1]

In contraceptive social marketing (CSM) programs, contraceptives are distributed at subsidized prices through existing retail outlets. The objectives are to make contraceptives more widely available, at lower cost, through a larger variety of locations, and with better hours of operation than previously. The CSM program acts to supplement other modes of delivery, giving consumers an added choice among the various channels of contraceptive supply.

COVERAGE

1. In some countries, an appreciable proportion of the urban population and even part of the rural population are covered at least to some extent by the CSM program.

   1.a. Observers in developing countries, estimating CSM coverage in broad ranges (*Table 1*), report that up to 25 percent of the urban or rural population (or both) is covered in nine of 23 responding countries, 25 to 50 percent is covered in seven countries, and above 50 percent is covered in eight countries.

Table 1 Percentage of urban and rural populations covered by social marketing programs in developing countries

Country	Year	% of urban population covered	% of rural population covered
Cameroon	1989	<25	<25
Ghana	1989	25–50	25–50
Zimbabwe	1989	<25	<25
Bolivia	1989	<25	<25
Colombia	1989	25–50	<25
Costa Rica	1989	>50	>50
Dominican Republic	1989	>50	25–50
El Salvador	1990	25–50	<25
Guatemala	1989	25–50	u
Honduras	1989	>50	25–50
Jamaica	1989	>50	25–50
Mexico	1989	25–50	25–50
Peru	1989	<25	u
Trinidad and Tobago	1989	>50	25–50
Egypt	1989	25–50	25–50
Morocco	1989	<25	u
Bangladesh	1989	>50	25–50
India	1989	<25	<25
Indonesia	1989	<25	<25
Nepal	1989	25–50	25–50
Pakistan	1989	<25	<25
Sri Lanka	1989	>50	>50
Taiwan	1986	98	94

u = unknown.
Source: Ross et al., 1992, Table 13. As explained there, detailed sources were 1987 and 1989 questionnaires sent to developing countries; SOMARC/The Futures Group, SOMARC II 1990 Sales Report, Washington, DC, courtesy of Sharon Tipping; and *Social Marketing Forum* (various issues). Other information came from J. Sherris, B. Ravenholt, and R. Blackburn, "Contraceptive Social Marketing: Lessons from Experience," *Population Reports* Series J, No. 30, July–August 1985.

EFFORT LEVELS

2. Countries have been distributed along a scale from zero to four according to the extent of the effort they give to their CSM programs. This scale is based upon the proportion of the total population that is covered by the CSM program. Many programs operate chiefly in the urban sector, which dilutes the score, but rural programs are included wherever they exist.

CSM Score	1982	1989
0–.99	88	67
1.0–1.99	4	9
2.0–2.99	3	9
3.0–3.99	0	7
4.0[a]	8	11
No. of countries	103	103

Source: Population Council Databank, 1992
[a] 4.0 is used for all values of 4.0 or above.

2.a. Most countries fall at low values, because they have not yet established a CSM program or because its coverage is still limited. Some countries fall at high values; the rest are at intermediate points.

2.b. Between 1982 and 1989, the distribution of scores shifted favorably, with 18 countries instead of eight at scores of three or above.

SALES AND CYP

3. Most CSM activity is concentrated in a few large countries, but some smaller countries do as well or better on a per capita basis.

3.a. Sales and CYP (couple-years of protection) results[2] for 44 countries (*Table 2*) show a disparate global picture: India's Nirodh program, which accounts for most of India's CYP, alone has one-third of all CYPs; Bangladesh has one-seventh and Egypt one-seventh. Next come Pakistan, at eight percent; Indo-

Table 2 Contraceptive social marketing sales summary: Sales/CYP data

Country and year	Orals	Condoms	Foam	Total CYP	Country and year	Orals	Condoms	Foam	Total CYP
Bangladesh					Indonesia				
1990	6,207,791	83,698,808	212,430	1,316,635	1990	745,772	5,858,381	—	115,951
1991	7,965,466	82,676,369	na	1,439,492	1991	1,153,321	5,928,956	—	148,007
Benin					Ivory Coast				
1990	—	382,364	—	3,824	1991	—	1,828,434	—	18,284
1991	—	633,932	—	6,339	Jamaica				
Bolivia					1990	525,672	1,792,516	—	58,361
1990	58,009	118,368	—	5,646	1991	546,218	1,917,852	—	61,195
1991	88,934	376,743	—	10,609	Jordan				
Brazil					1990	—	334,095	—	3,341
1991	—	405,504	—	4,055	1991	—	115,488	—	1,155
Burkina Faso					Kenya				
1991	—	2,794,952	—	27,950	1990	na	300,714	—	3,007
Burundi					1991	2,677	497,884	—	5,185
1990	—	94,000	—	940	Malawi				
1991	—	164,984	—	1,650	1991	—	159,416	—	1,594
Cameroon					Malaysia				
1990	—	1,990,255	—	19,903	1991	—	823,540	—	8,235
1991	—	3,193,996	—	31,940	Mexico				
Central African Republic					1990	—	3,974,688	—	39,747
1991	—	310,080	—	3,101	1991	—	5,579,393	—	55,794
Colombia					Morocco				
1990	5,444,480	6,407,785	3,006,656	512,951	1990	—	1,053,669	—	10,537
1991	5,973,632	6,319,715	2,163,276	544,360	1991	—	1,774,809	—	17,748
Costa Rica					Nepal				
1990	—	2,330,515	—	23,305	1990	190,869	2,947,323	486,864	49,024
1991	—	2,937,152	—	29,372	1991	247,853	4,422,651	671,796	70,010
Dominican Republic					Nigeria				
1990	579,910	449,547	—	49,104	1990	—	1,131,582	—	11,316
1991	497,579	869,016	—	46,965	1991	—	1,876,129	—	18,761
Eastern Caribbean					Pakistan				
1990	—	121,839	na	1,218	1990	—	73,835,136	—	738,351
1991	—	90,399	na	904	1991	—	73,385,375	—	733,854
Ecuador					Papua New Guinea				
1990	585,570	na	—	45,044	1991	—	94,317	—	943
1991	716,792	214,305	—	57,281	Peru				
Egypt					1991	592,926	—	1,842,924	64,039
1990	2,082,434	17,057,744	—	330,765	Philippines				
1991	2,011,655	14,668,488	—	301,428	1990	—	201,744	—	2,017
El Salvador					1991	—	1,266,048	—	12,660
1990	296,540	1,807,056	—	40,881	Sri Lanka				
1991	287,345	1,769,372	—	39,797	1990	547,628	5,664,125	76,593	99,532
Ethiopia					1991	655,722	6,766,566	80,697	118,913
1990	—	699,506	—	6,995	Thailand				
1991	—	3,782,454	—	37,825	1991	814,327	—	—	62,641
Ghana					Trinidad				
1990	452,444	3,586,500	1,602,200	86,690	1990	—	209,288	—	2,093
1991	435,300	3,748,300	1,909,400	90,062	1991	—	208,149	—	2,081
Guatemala					Turkey				
1990	170,234	1,321,857	608,500	32,398	1991	—	4,469,430	—	44,694
1991	183,460	1,600,464	589,656	36,014	Uganda				
Guinea					1991	—	302,106	—	3,021
1991	—	140,236	—	1,402	Zaire				
Haiti					1990	—	7,898,413	1,658,880	95,573
1990	10,215	357,139	—	4,357	1991	—	18,301,507	1,947,208	202,487
1991	37,464	576,513	—	8,647	Zimbabwe				
Honduras					1990	43,793	769,420	—	11,063
1990	248,280	739,722	—	26,496	1991	67,033	1,182,083	—	16,977
1991	215,788	599,912	—	22,598	Total global CYPs				
India					1990	—	—	—	3,747,065
1991	164,525	327,199,600	—	3,284,652	1991	—	—	—	7,694,721

na = not available
Note: One CYP equals 13 cycles of pills, 100 condoms, or 100 foaming tablets.
Sources: DKI International, *Family Planning World* 2(3), May/June 1992 and John Stover, personal communication.

Figure 1 CYPs as percentage of target market[a]

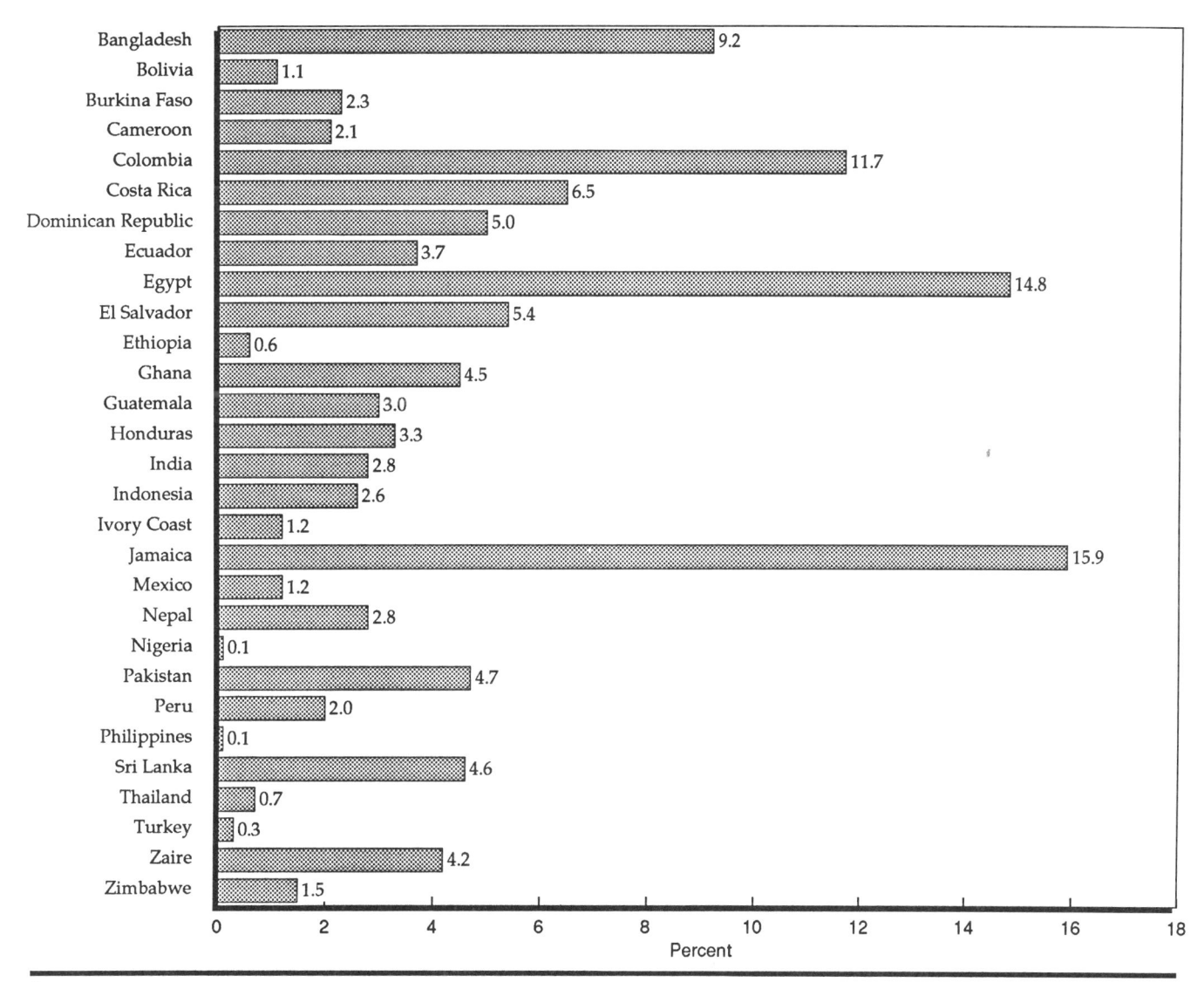

Country	Percent
Bangladesh	9.2
Bolivia	1.1
Burkina Faso	2.3
Cameroon	2.1
Colombia	11.7
Costa Rica	6.5
Dominican Republic	5.0
Ecuador	3.7
Egypt	14.8
El Salvador	5.4
Ethiopia	0.6
Ghana	4.5
Guatemala	3.0
Honduras	3.3
India	2.8
Indonesia	2.6
Ivory Coast	1.2
Jamaica	15.9
Mexico	1.2
Nepal	2.8
Nigeria	0.1
Pakistan	4.7
Peru	2.0
Philippines	0.1
Sri Lanka	4.6
Thailand	0.7
Turkey	0.3
Zaire	4.2
Zimbabwe	1.5

[a]Target market calculated as 80 percent of women in union, ages 15–44.
Source: DKT International, "1991 Contraceptive Social Marketing Statistics," June 1992.

nesia, at eight percent; and Colombia, at seven percent: The other programs, some in small countries, have trivial proportions of the total. However, these may amount to appreciable proportions of their own populations, as in Jamaica and elsewhere (below).

3.b. Measured against their own population sizes, the size of programs still varies widely (*Figure 1*), but Jamaica, Costa Rica, the Dominican Republic, and El Salvador fall at higher points here than in *Table 2*. The range is from 0.1 to 16 percent of women in union (taken as 80 percent of all women of reproductive age); measured in this way, the median value in *Figure 1* is only 2.8 percent, but seven countries are above 5 percent and three are above 10 percent.

The reference to 80 percent of women in union is a severe and inappropriate standard in some countries, since the program may focus only on the urban sector or on part of the country. In fact, some CSM programs now direct their marketing campaigns to carefully selected income groups that are neither the very poor, who cannot pay, nor the well-to-do, who need no subsidization. Of five income-level groups from well off through poor, the focus is on members of the two middle-income groups who desire spacing methods.

SUBSTITUTION

4. In countries with high contraceptive prevalence, CSM programs may partially substitute for other supply sources, attracting current users who are simply switching from another source. However, in countries with low contraceptive prevalence, CSM programs do not appear to compete appreciably with other contraceptive suppliers (Sherris et al., 1985; Binnendijk, 1986). Marketing strategies are used to minimize substitution for the commercial sector (Stover, 1993a).

4.a. Projects in Kenya, Bangladesh, and Nepal found that CSM programs offer little competition to public and private sector programs. However, the CSM programs in Sri Lanka, Thailand, and Colombia (all countries with high prevalence) may have reduced private sector sales (Sheon et al., 1987).

4.b. In Bangladesh most contraceptives are supplied by the government program. As the supplies provided by the CSM program grew, the number of contraceptives supplied by all programs grew by the same amount, suggesting little switching (Sherris et al., 1985).

4.c. Switching from free government supplies to CSM sources reduces the public burden and amounts to partial cost recovery from sales income.

4.d. Programs that are directed primarily at higher income clients probably encounter more switching, since many such clients may have been buying at regular commercial prices (Sherris et al., 1985). However, CSM programs may still improve the availability of supplies for such clients if commercial outlets have been inactive.

4.e. A review of eight CSM programs (*Table 3*) found that about 25 to 50 percent of customers were new users, with the rest divided between switchers and others, in unclear proportions. (Some "previous users" may have been nonusers for some time prior to buying supplies from the CSM program.)

MANAGEMENT FEATURES

5. CSM program experience has yielded certain management guidelines; however, no one management structure is appropriate for every country. The strategy chosen must fit the local circumstances.

5.a. Several different CSM structures are used; programs are managed by various agencies (Sherris et al., 1985; Sheon et al., 1987). Examples:

* a family planning association (Colombia, Sri Lanka, El Salvador, and Honduras)
* private sector organizations established solely for that purpose (Nepal, Mexico, Thailand, and Guatemala)
* semi-autonomous or quasi-governmental agencies, governed by a board or council (Bangladesh and Egypt)
* government agencies (India and Jamaica)
* an established commercial distributor (Caribbean).

5.b. CSM programs operate in a complex institutional environment; they are exposed to difficulties that often arise in the unpredictable interplay of government, donors, and the commercial world. Multiple agreements must be negotiated and kept, special permissions are needed, and the business venture must succeed. Whatever management strategy is adopted, communication and coordination with relevant government agencies are vital. In the initial stages of a program, technical experts are an important link between host governments, donor agencies, and CSM management (Sherris et al., 1985).

PRICING

6. Two goals conflict in setting CSM prices: low cost versus program sustainability. Certain guidelines have emerged:

6.a. In setting prices, a year's supply should cost less than 1 percent of the yearly household income of lower income groups; prices should be comparable to those of other commonly purchased household commodities (such as soap). Further, prices should be approximately half the cost of other commercially available contraceptives (Binnendijk, 1985; Sherris et al., 1985; Sheon et al., 1987).

6.b. Prices should be low enough so that all potential customers can afford them, but not so low as to imply poor quality (Sherris et al., 1985). In Thailand, many women experiencing side effects from a low-cost brand of pills switched to a higher priced brand, under the assumption that the higher price implied higher quality.

6.c. Prices of products should rise with inflation. Generally, sales are unaffected by small price in-

Table 3 Previous use of family planning among current customers of social marketing programs, as reported in customer surveys, 1986–1990

Method and country	Year	Number surveyed	New users of family planning(%)	Previous users of same method by type of previous source - Subsidized	Commercial	Other[a]	Previous users of other methods
Oral contraceptives							
Dominican Republic	1986–87	(252)	34	13	40	0	13
Honduras	1986	(222)[b]	na	49	41	10	na
Peru	1989	(362)	53[c]	——— 13 ———		2	32[d]
Condoms							
Barbados	1989	(140)	31	9	27	0	31
Ghana	1990	(249)	43	7	3	3	44[d]
Indonesia	1988	(101)[e]	26	0	40	0	34
Mexico	1988	(388)	32	33[f]	21[f]	0	17
Morocco	1990	(242)	40	na	na	na	na

na = not available.
[a] Source not identifiable as either subsidized or commercial, or source unknown.
[b] Previous oral contraceptive users only.
[c] Includes 19 percent who had used traditional methods.
[d] May include previous users of other social marketing products.
[e] Ever-users of Dua Lima condoms.
[f] May include multiple responses. Row adds to 103%.
Source: Lande and Geller, 1991, Table 3.

creases but are reduced by large increases. Thus, to avoid a drop in sales, prices should be increased slowly over time (Sherris et al., 1985), especially for condoms, since their sales tend to respond more directly to prices than do pill sales (Boone et al., 1985). In El Salvador's program, a 100 percent increase in prices was blamed for a 50 percent decline in sales (Sheon, 1987).

6.d. Price mark-ups should be high enough to encourage distributors, wholesalers, and retailers (Sherris et al., 1985). However, the original price must be modest enough so that after these mark-ups, the final price to the consumer will be attractively low.

PROMOTION

7. **CSM programs actively promote and advertise their products, especially condoms and pills.**

   7.a. Radio and TV, as well as other media, have been used to promote contraceptives to large audiences. Promotion campaigns have had four objectives: to draw attention to the products by brand name, to create a product image for the intended submarket (young people, couples, and so on), to inform the audience about how the product works and how to use it, and to tell clients where to get the product and what it costs (Sherris et al., 1985).

   7.b. In most countries, condom promotions have emphasized their safety, effectiveness, and appropriateness for married couples, to overcome their poor image (Sherris et al., 1985).

   7.c. Person-to-person promotion and education are important to educate retailers and health care providers about the product and to stimulate interest in the CSM program (Sherris et al., 1985; Schellstede and Ciszewski, 1984).

   7.d. Promotion efforts need to be both extensive and continuous, and any governmental or public objections to program advertising will probably lessen over time. Hiring an experienced advertising agency may be the most cost-effective way of promoting the products (Sherris et al., 1985).

   7.e. Promotion costs are often the largest item in a CSM budget. India's CSM program spent approximately 75 percent of its budget on advertising, and Egypt spent over one-third on it (Sherris et al., 1985; Sheon, 1987).

COST-EFFECTIVENESS

8. **Several factors affect the cost-effectiveness of CSM programs (Binnendijk, 1986; Sherris et al., 1985).**

   8.a. Programs tend to have high costs in the first year of operation, and then to become more cost-effective (*Figure 2*). This reflects low initial sales and high start-

Figure 2 Cost per couple-year of protection, selected developing countries

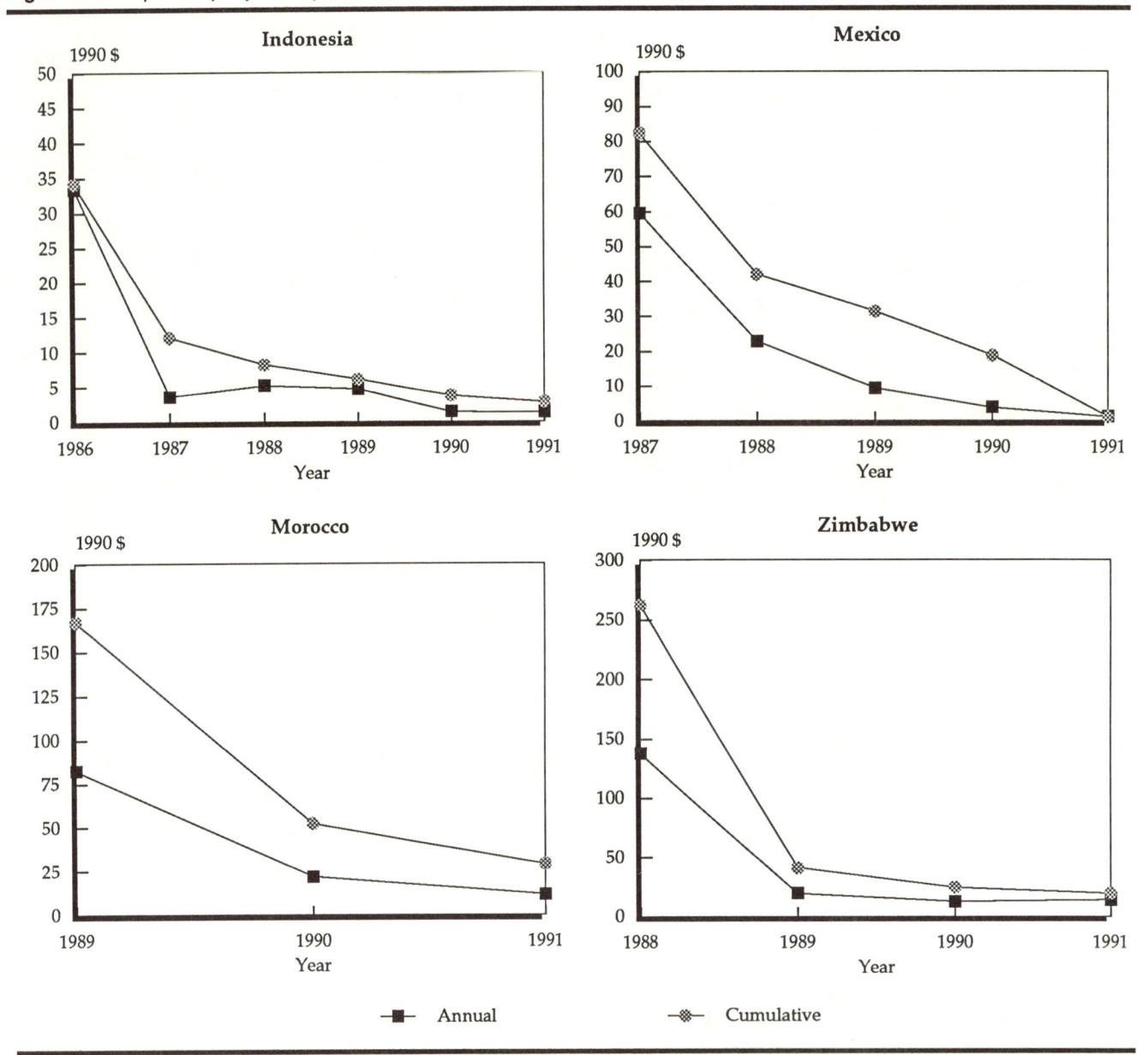

*[Four line charts showing Annual and Cumulative cost per couple-year of protection in 1990 $ for:
- Indonesia (1986–1991)
- Mexico (1987–1991)
- Morocco (1989–1991)
- Zimbabwe (1988–1991)]*

■ Annual   ✦ Cumulative

Source: Stover, 1993b.

up costs, such as recruiting and training staff, launching an advertising campaign, and contacting retail outlets to inform them about the CSM venture. "Not all these costs continue into future years of the project," and as sales increase, "... the costs are divided by a larger number of CYP provided (Stover and Wagman, 1992).

8.b. Early delays may occur that reduce sales while fixed costs remain. Changes in program management, in government policies and regulations, and in the economic and international environment, as well as other factors, can all cause delays.

8.c. Programs whose main objective is to reach as many couples as possible tend to be less cost-efficient than those that target clear subgroups and seek some degree of self-sufficiency.

8.d. Cost-effectiveness is influenced by the general level of development and economic conditions. Costs of commodities, labor, and other program inputs vary by country, as do such infrastructural aspects as the ease of transport, media coverage of the population, communication facilities, and banking systems.

8.e. Programs with high sales volumes tend to have lower costs per unit sold. Condom sales tend to respond primarily to marketing activities, including price levels and advertising, whereas oral sales tend to respond more to social and economic conditions, including level of income and education, and communication systems. Oral sales also increase as prescription requirements decline. Program duration is an important predictor of both oral and condom sales rates (Boone et al., 1985; Sherris et al., 1985; Sheon et al., 1987).

8.f. Because CSM programs use existing commercial channels and have no clinical facilities or medical personnel, they appear to cost much less than other delivery systems. A comparison of 63 projects in 10 countries put their average cost per CYP at about US $2.00, compared with about US $13.00 for a regular clinic service and about US $14.00 for community-based distribution programs (Huber and Harvey, 1989).

8.g. All cost calculations are subject to qualifications. Most CSM programs receive substantial donor support to make subsidized prices possible, contraceptive supplies are often imported free of charge to the program, and different cost calculations treat such items differently.

8.h. Costs to donors and local governments depend upon the CSM model employed. Over the years a partial evolution has occurred, shifting certain types of costs away from the donors and to the local implementing organizations. Contraceptive commodities can be obtained more cheaply from local sources, or can be purchased commercially by the project itself. Existing local companies can implement the project and distribute the products, instead of creating new infrastructures from donor funds. Finally, a CSM project may be entirely operated and financed as an indigenous activity, with the donor contribution devoted only to all or part of the advertising and promotion costs. These features help to contain the donor role to the start-up phase, with a declining burden through time, and thereby enhance the sustainability of the CSM activity (Stover, 1993a and 1993b).

NOTES

1. An early draft of this chapter was prepared by Marjorie Rich, formerly of the Population Council staff.
2. Four measures are used to measure the results of CSM programs: sales, couple-years of protection (CYPs), cost per CYP, and coverage estimates. *Sales data* are generally easy to obtain, but usually only at the distributor, wholesaler, and/or retailer levels, not at the consumer level. This impairs most estimates of what percentage of products actually reach (and are used by) the consumer. Both CYP and cost per CYP are calculated from sales data, thus they usually reflect any inaccuracies inherent in the sales data. *Couple-years of protection* uses the quantity of each method needed to protect one couple for one year. For pills, this is generally assumed to be 13 cycles. For condoms and spermicides, it is usually 100 units. Some programs have estimated the conversion to be as high as 150 condoms or spermicides for each CYP, reflecting a different estimate of coital frequency or an allowance for wastage. *Cost per CYP* is calculated by dividing the total cost of running the program by the total CYP obtained. Cost calculations have their own problems; also, not all programs measure cost the same way: For example, some include donated contraceptives, technical assistance, and so on, while others do not. *Coverage estimates* include the percentage of MWRA, or alternatively all users, in the country who obtain their supplies from the CSM program. The latter measure reflects not only the action of the CSM program, but also the availability of contraceptives from other sources as well.

REFERENCES

Binnendijk, A. L. 1986. "AID's experience with contraceptive social marketing: A synthesis of project evaluation findings." *AID Evaluation Special Study* No. 40, USAID.

Boone, M. S., J. U. Farley, and S. J. Samuel. 1985. "A cross-country study of commercial contraceptive sales programs: Factors that lead to success." *Studies in Family Planning* 16(1):30–39.

Cherris, J., B. Ravenholt, and R. Blackburn. 1985. "Contraceptive Social Marketing: Lessons from Experience," *Population Reports* Series J, No. 30, July-August 1985.

Huber, S. C. and P. D. Harvey. 1989. "Family planning programs in ten developing countries: Cost effectiveness by mode of service delivery." *Biosocial Science* 21(3):267–277.

Lande, R.E. and J. S. Geller. 1991. "Paying for family planning." *Population Reports* Series J, Number 39, November.

Ross, J., W.P. Mauldin, S.R. Green, E.R. Cooke. 1992. *Family Planning and Child Survival Programs as Assessed in 1991*. New York: The Population Council.

Schellstede, W. P. and R. L. Ciszewski. 1984. "Social marketing of contraceptives in Bangladesh." *Studies in Family Planning* 15(1):30–39.

Sheon, A., W.P. Schellstede, and B. Derr. 1987. "Contraceptive social marketing." In *Organizing for Effective Family Planning Programs*. R.J. Lapham and G.B. Simmons, eds. Washington, DC: National Academy Press.

Sherris, J. D., B. B. Ravenholt, and R. Blackburn. 1985. "Contraceptive social marketing: Lessons and experience." *Population Reports* 13(2).

Stover, J. 1993a. Personal communication.

Stover, J. 1993b. "The contribution of contraceptive social marketing programs to the sustainability of family planning services." Paper presented at the 1993 annual meeting of the Population Association of America, Cincinnati, April.

Stover, J. and A. Wagman. 1992. *The Costs of Contraceptive Social Marketing Programs Implemented Through the SOMARC Project*. Special Study #1, June.

Chapter 5

POSTPARTUM PROGRAMS[1]

One mode of delivering family planning services is the postpartum program, initiated in the late 1960s through a special international demonstration effort (Zatuchni, 1970; Castadot et al., 1975). The concept is to offer women information and services at three points of contact: at the prenatal visit, at the time of delivery, and at the six-week checkup. Outpatient family planning services are included for all couples regardless of interval since birth, as are postabortal services. In practice, many hospitals and maternity homes omit one or more of these features, or omit some contraceptive methods.

The advantages of postpartum programs include:

* The logistics are simple—adding family planning to already established maternity services is convenient for women and efficient for administration.

* They offer a low-cost means of extending family planning services over a few years to much of the active childbearing population, especially in urban areas. Startup costs are low, as are marginal operating costs; costs are also low compared to those of other delivery modes.

* They can advance health objectives by raising attendance at the six-week checkup, increasing infant immunizations, reducing the frequency of short birth intervals with their severe dangers to infant survival, reducing the frequency both of repeat septic abortions and of unwanted births, and raising the proportion of births that are attended through the attraction of contraceptive services in the maternity facility.

* They can avert many unwanted conceptions by providing contraceptives promptly after an abortion or birth, since the most fecund couples tend to conceive quickly again, before obtaining contraceptive protection. This applies especially to those who breastfeed partially or not at all.

The disadvantages of postpartum programs include:

* Certain hormonal methods are not medically appropriate soon after birth (though they are after abortion). In particular, estrogen-based pills reduce the quantity of breastmilk and pass steroids on to the infant. Appropriate hormonal methods are the progestin-based ones, such as the injectable, the minipill, and NORPLANT®.

* Historically, most postpartum programs have been urban-based and in established medical facilities; consequently, large rural populations have been relatively neglected (exceptions noted below).

* A full postpartum program requires coordination among several departments of a hospital: prenatal, delivery, abortion care, surgery (for sterilization), and multiple outpatient departments, especially where family planning and maternal and child health (MCH) are separate. Also, overtaxed medical facilities sometimes defer family planning services, including sterilization, viewing them as elective procedures.

COVERAGE AND POTENTIAL

1. **In many countries a substantial proportion of births are now attended by medical personnel, though variation across countries is still considerable.**

   1.a. In more than half of developing countries (51 of 96), over 50 percent of births are attended by health personnel in established institutions (*Table 1*). In about a third, over 70 percent of births are attended. Still, the proportion of births that are attended varies greatly by country, from less than 10 percent to over 90 percent. Further, variation among countries is large within each of four regions.

   1.b. Trained health personnel in many countries see substantial proportions of women either prenatally, at delivery, or postnatally, thus providing ready occasions for dispensing family planning advice and services. The following findings (Thapa et al. 1992) document the potential for providing services around the time of birth.

   Prenatal: In 25 countries with DHS surveys, over 80 percent of pregnant women were seen prenatally in

Table 1 Distribution of 96 developing countries by the percentage of all deliveries occurring in hospitals and maternity centers

Percent	Asia	Latin America	Middle East/ North Africa	Sub-Saharan Africa	Total
0–9	4	0	0	3	7
10–19	3	0	2	2	7
20–29	2	2	2	6	12
30–39	2	1	1	5	9
40–49	0	2	0	8	10
50–59	2	2	1	4	9
60–69	2	3	3	4	12
70–79	0	0	1	4	5
80–89	6	4	2	2	14
90–100	1	8	2	0	11
Total	(22)	(22)	(14)	(38)	(96)

Note: World Bank figures for 1985, covering 61 developing countries, give a similar percentage distribution in the total column above. See World Bank, 1992, Table 28, based upon WHO and UNICEF country information.
Source: Population Council Databank, 1992.

12 countries, and over 50 percent in 19.

At delivery: Over 70 percent of women were attended at delivery in nine countries, and over 50 percent in 12. In general, this distribution is somewhat less favorable than for prenatal visits.

Postnatal: The available information pertains to contacts with trained health personnel for at least one immunization. Over 70 percent of women report such a contact in 10 countries, and over 50 percent in 14, out of 21 surveys that included the question. These data are suggestive of the family planning potential, even though immunization services are often not linked to family planning services. Closer linkage of various MCH services is a common need.

2. Many countries provide a family planning information and education service in delivery facilities.

   2.a. Respondents from 76 of the 96 countries in *Table 1* reported that a family planning information and education service exists for women delivering in hos-

Table 2 Distribution of 76 countries by percentage of women delivering in hospitals and maternity centers who receive the family planning information service

Percent	Asia	Latin America	Middle East/ North Africa	Sub-Saharan Africa	Total
0–9	2	2	2	8	14
10–19	0	2	1	6	9
20–29	3	4	2	3	12
30–39	0	1	1	4	6
40–49	1	3	0	2	6
50–59	1	0	1	4	6
60–69	0	2	1	1	4
70–79	4	1	0	0	5
80–89	2	4	1	0	7
90–100	3	2	0	2	7
Total	(16)	(21)	(9)	(30)	(76)

Source: Population Council Databank, 1992.

pitals and maternity centers (*Table 2*) (this is the only available global estimate). Coverage varies greatly: The proportion of delivering women who receive the service varies from less than 10 percent in 14 countries to over 90 percent in seven. Even sub-Saharan countries are distributed broadly: While over half fall below 30 percent coverage, about one-third fall above 40 percent coverage.

UNMET NEED

3. **The failure to obtain contraception soon after giving birth contributes to the unmet need for family planning. At 7–9 months after giving birth, many women are exposed to pregnancy who do not wish to become pregnant but who still have not obtained contraceptive protection.**

   3.a. Among women in union who were interviewed 7–9 months after a birth in 25 DHS surveys, a subgroup was "exposed": not pregnant and not abstaining, with menses having returned. Among women in this group who were not using contraceptives, substantial percentages did not want another child or did not want one soon. As *Table 3* shows, these percentages ranged to very high levels. The base varies, that is, the proportions of exposed women who were not using contraceptives tend to be quite high in Africa and lower elsewhere, but these remarkably high figures show much unmet need among this group, whose menses have resumed. Other women had already become pregnant by 7–9 months postpartum; those are omitted here (Thapa et al., 1992).

4. **Substantial proportions of women who give birth conceive again within nine months, and more do so within 15 months (*Table 4*), leading to short birth intervals that elevate the mortality risks for both infants. (See Chapter 10 for further discussion of this topic.) To alleviate this contraceptive services are needed early, especially for the more fecund couples, at highest risk of an unwanted conception.**

   Table 4 contains more than one birth for many reporting women, since the data cover up to 15 years experience. Thus, women with more births close together contribute more to the table, and they are the ones with multiple infants at higher risks. Some brief intervals are produced by early infant deaths, with abbreviated lactation. (The following figures are from Hobcraft, 1991, based on 25 DHS surveys.)

5. **Many women become pregnant sooner after a previous birth than they desire.**

Table 3 Percentage of noncontracepting women in union exposed to the risk of pregnancy 7–9 months after a birth, who want no more children or want none soon

Region and country	% of noncontracepting exposed women who want to stop or space
Sub-Saharan Africa	
Burundi	94
Ghana	88
Kenya	79
Togo	77
Senegal	67
Botswana	63
Mali	59
Uganda	55
Liberia	41
North Africa	
Tunisia	80
Morocco	80
Egypt	66
Latin America	
Colombia	95
Peru	90
Ecuador	90
Dominican Republic	86
Bolivia	83
Guatemala	82
Trinidad and Tobago	81
Brazil	73
Mexico	64
Asia	
Sri Lanka	89
Thailand	84
Indonesia	76

Note: In the sub-Saharan and North African countries, as well as in the three Asian countries, a majority of these noncontraceptors want to space; in most of Latin America, a majority want to stop.
Source: Thapa et al., 1992.

5.a. Only 11 percent (average) of respondents in 25 DHS surveys wanted their next birth to come within two years of their previous one, but 35 percent had birth intervals that were shorter than two years (Hobcraft, 1991, Table 11; Westoff, 1991, Table 4.1). In every country the difference between the actual and desired birth-interval length was very large. Also, these data omit unwanted early pregnancies that end in induced abortion.

Table 4 Percentage of births conceived early (within nine months or 15 months of a previous birth), by region

	Number of	Percent	
Region	countries	≤9 months[a]	≤15 months[b]
Latin America	(9)	17–30	36–47
North Africa	(3)	18–24	37–41
Sub-Saharan Africa	(10)	7–20	20–37
Asia	(3)	14–15	30–31
Mean	25 DHS surveys	17	35
	18 WFS surveys	22	42

[a] Birth interval 17.9 months or less.
[b] Birth interval 23.9 months or less.
Note: Some births were 1–2 months premature, so conceptions occurred later than indicated.
Source: Hobcraft, 1991.

CURRENT METHOD RECOMMENDATIONS

6. Currently, health officials in many countries suggest that breastfeeding mothers initiate contraceptive use within about four months of giving birth (before 18 weeks), that is, before weaning would normally occur, and some recommend it within the first six weeks (*Table 5*). Such recommendations, when implemented for the appropriate methods, help protect against another pregnancy for those who breastfeed partially or not at all.

6.a. However, many officials recommend otherwise, contrary to the best international standards. In nine countries the recommendations are to start pill use (not differentiated by type) too early, and for the IUD, too late. Country variation is considerable (generally on the late side) for condoms, injectables, and sterilization, with no consistent differences by region (not shown).

In general, estrogen-based methods are inadvisable at any time during lactation. Barrier methods may be used at any time, and sterilization can occur at any time (and vasectomy for the spouse even during pregnancy). IUD insertion can occur at any time. The expulsion rate is higher when insertion occurs very soon after birth, but among delivering women who desire the IUD some would return for it later whereas others would find it difficult to do so; therefore, the decision on an early insertion is a matter of judgment.

INTEREST IN POSTPARTUM SERVICES

7. Interest in postpartum services has been substantial in many countries.

7.a. There is extensive behavioral evidence that many women desire contraceptive assistance at or soon af-

Table 5 Number of weeks postpartum that breastfeeding mothers are advised to start using contraception, by method, 86 developing countries

	Weeks postpartum					Number of
Method	≤5	6–11	12–17	≤17	18+	countries
Pills	9	20	9	38	15	(53)
Injectables	1	13	8	22	10	(32)
IUD	8	26	9	43	16	(59)
Barrier/condom	9	18	4	31	11	(42)
Spermicides	1	5	2	8	3	(11)
Sterilization	0	4	3	7	5	(12)

Note: For 86 developing countries; not all countries replied for each method.
Source: Population Council Databank, from 1989 questionnaire survey to country informants.

ter birth, as do many who present at hospitals with incomplete abortions. As early as the 1966–73 period, when contraceptive options were more limited than now, large-scale postpartum programs experienced substantial response rates. The 138 hospitals participating in the International Postpartum Program during those years saw 3.5 million obstetric cases (including women presenting with incomplete abortions). Some 1.1 million women adopted contraception through the program, most of them before leaving the hospital or within three months afterwards; the others came for service after a longer delay, or they heard about the program by word of mouth without having been a patient at one of the hospitals. As an average over the 21 countries involved, the ratio of contraceptive adopters to the obstetric volume was nearly one to three. This substantial response encouraged widespread adoption of the postpartum approach, both in maternity services and in outpatient clinics (Castadot et al., 1975; Zatuchni, 1970).

7.b. Motivation for postpartum contraception appears in results from a uniform series of small studies in six countries, based on 100 to 110 respondents in each country: Colombia, Dominican Republic, India, Kenya, Mali, and Turkey (Landry et al., 1992). Mean values across all sites, for women interviewed before leaving the hospital, were as follows: 43 percent had ever used a method, and 20 percent had been using a method when they became accidentally pregnant. Fifteen percent took a method before leaving the hospital, an additional 29 percent stated they intended to begin use within six weeks, and a further 34 percent, within six months, for a total of 78 percent starting or intending to start use within six months. Forty-nine percent said they did not want the last pregnancy either at that time or ever, and 55 percent said they now want no more children.

7.c. Motivation for early contraception is evident in a Peruvian experiment. A variety of contraceptive methods were offered prior to discharge to women who delivered in one ward, and 81 percent accepted a method before leaving the hospital. Women who delivered in a control ward that received no in-hospital contraceptive services also adopted contraceptive methods at an appreciable rate soon after leaving the hospital; interviews at six months found 82 percent of the experimental group using a method and 69 percent of the control group doing so. Thus, substantial, early contraceptive practice was found in both groups, with somewhat more in the experimental group. Approximately 50 percent of subjects were lost to follow-up, but both groups had equivalent non-respondent characteristics (Foreit et al., 1993; Population Council, 1992).

7.d. Among current users of sterilization in 16 of 18 countries studied in DHS surveys, over 30 percent had taken the method postpartum; in 10 of these countries, over half had done so (Rutenberg and Landry, 1991).

EFFECTS UPON ABORTIONS

8. **Some facilities that offer postpartum or postabortion contraception have experienced a decline in the number of septic abortion cases seen.**

8.a. In the International Postpartum Program, hospitals experienced a decline in the monthly number of abortion cases, with a 10 percent fall from the three-year average prior to the postpartum program to the period 18–24 months later. A similar comparison over time for six US hospitals showed a 22 percent decline, though with an irregular time trend (Zatuchni, 1970).

8.b. Analysis of individual hospitals showed considerable variation: 10 hospitals experienced declines in septic abortion cases from 18–41 percent, five experienced an increase, and nine showed no clear change. Some evidence suggested that declines in the number of abortion cases partly reflected the general availability of family planning services in the area (Zatuchni, 1970, pp. 69–74), as well as other factors, in addition to the impact of the hospitals' own postpartum and postabortion services.

BREASTFEEDING AS A CONTRACEPTIVE METHOD

9. **Breastfeeding lengthens the birth interval, on average, but is only partially useful for the individual as a contraceptive strategy, and it has limited programmatic potential as a substitute for contraceptive methods.**

9.a. On a population basis, extended breastfeeding depresses the fertility rate (Bongaarts, 1975); however, except under special circumstances, it is no guarantee for the individual woman. Pregnancies can occur during the early months of breastfeeding, and even before the return of menses. In one study, ovulation occurred before the menses returned in 20 percent of women who were bottlefeeding their babies and in 45 percent of women who were breastfeeding (Howie et al., cited in Winikoff and Mensch, 1991, p. 295).

9.b. The strict practice of breastfeeding for the first six months after birth has been examined as a deliberate contraceptive option. "More than 98 percent protection from pregnancy in the first six months" is promised if two conditions are met: that breastfeeding is full or nearly full, and that amenorrhea continues. If either condition is compromised, other means are then needed to retain a high degree of protection (FHI, 1988; Kennedy et al., 1989). The report says that women relying on breastfeeding for its contraceptive efficacy should delay introduction of other foods, although it also notes that these are usually needed between the fourth and sixth months.

9.c. Full breastfeeding, in any case is very uncommon, as *Figure 1* makes clear. This is unfortunate, and even though many countries are trying to encourage breastfeeding, actual practice falls far short of giving protection against unwanted pregnancy. The brevity of full breastfeeding limits its protective effect, and contraceptive supplementation is required if unmet need is to be addressed.

9.d. Despite its fallibility as a contraceptive for the individual, breastfeeding greatly enhances infant health; moreover, it does not appear to be in decline in the developing world at large. In their careful assessment of breastfeeding data in WFS and DHS surveys for 47 countries, Trussell and colleagues (1992) found that breastfeeding durations have not changed markedly. They are somewhat longer in some countries and somewhat shorter in some others. They are consistently longer among less educated and rural women, and they are increasing among urban women. Durations are clearly longer in Africa and Asia than in Latin America.

THE OVERLAP QUESTION

10. Early contraceptive use is advisable even though some of it overlaps with postpartum amenorrhea.

10.a. When breastfeeding confers reliable protection against pregnancy, simultaneous contraceptive use is thought to be redundant. However, several considerations qualify this. Much breastfeeding gives incomplete protection, as does some contraception. A programmatic emphasis on breastfeeding alone will result in unwanted pregnancies, yet breastfeeding is needed quite apart from its contraceptive effects. Programs that avoid overlapping protection by trying to delay contraception until the return of each woman's menses will not work well, since field programs cannot be so closely fine tuned. As with breast-

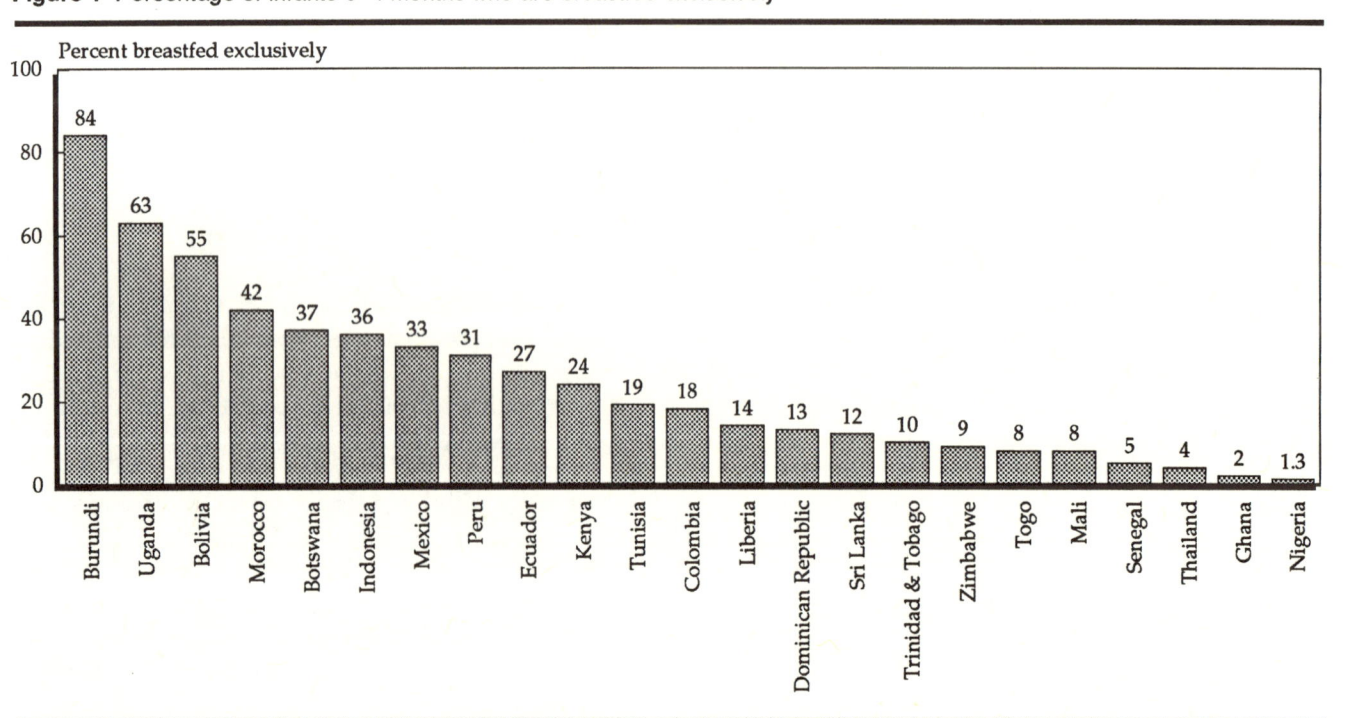

Figure 1 Percentage of infants 0–4 months who are breastfed exclusively

Country	Percent
Burundi	84
Uganda	63
Bolivia	55
Morocco	42
Botswana	37
Indonesia	36
Mexico	33
Peru	31
Ecuador	27
Kenya	24
Tunisia	19
Colombia	18
Liberia	14
Dominican Republic	13
Sri Lanka	12
Trinidad & Tobago	10
Zimbabwe	9
Togo	8
Mali	8
Senegal	5
Thailand	4
Ghana	2
Nigeria	1.3

Source: Ross et al., 1992, Figure 8; see also Table 35. Taken from DHS surveys.

feeding alone, such a strategy will cause unwanted pregnancies. It involves the risk of what has been termed "underlap," i.e., a gap between postpartum ovulation and the initiation of contraception.

10.b. Many women want contraceptive services (including sterilization) after delivery, while they are still at the facility (see 7.c.); indeed, some explicitly choose a facility for delivery that will provide contraception simultaneously. Overlap is a trivial consideration with sterilization, and is minor for the better IUDs, since the duration of overlap with full breastfeeding is a small part of their total protection time. Further, there are acceptable personal trade-offs with overlap: Women can initiate protection when they wish rather than having to wait; in addition, early access to condoms is needed as a measure against AIDS and other sexually transmitted diseases (STDs).

10.c. All these considerations underlie the provision of contraceptive advice and services, along with breastfeeding instruction, at all three points of contact: the prenatal visit, delivery, and the six-week checkup.

NOTES

1. This chapter is based partially upon draft materials prepared by Steven R. Green.
2. A response of "six weeks" is included in the "6–11 week" category. A response of "three months" is included in the "12–17" week category.
3. Column totals are not shown because the same respondent could reply to several items.
4. Data are only approximate; respondents within the same country often gave differing responses.

REFERENCES

Bongaarts, J. 1975. "Why high birth rates are so low." *Population and Development Review* 1(2):289–296.

Castadot, R. G. et al. 1975. "The international postpartum family planning program: Eight years of experience." *Reports on Population/Family Planning*, No. 18.

Family Health International. 1988. "Consensus statement: Breastfeeding as a family planning method." *The Lancet* Vol. II, No. 8621, November 19, pp.1,204–1,205.

Foreit, K., J.R. Foreit, G. Lagos, and A. Guzman. 1993. "Effectiveness and cost-effectiveness of postpartum IUD insertion in Lima, Peru" *International Family Planning Perspectives* 19(1):19–24.

Hobcraft, J. 1991. "Child spacing and child mortality." *Demographic and Health Surveys World Conference, August 5–7, 1991, Proceedings*, Vol. II:1,157–1,181. Columbia, Maryland: Institute for Resource Development/Macro Systems Inc.

Kennedy, K. I., R. Rivera, and A. S. McNeilly. 1989. "Consensus statement on the use of breastfeeding as a family planning method." *Contraception* 39(5):447–496.

Landry, E., C.S. Verme, L.M. Rabinovitz, and M. Geetanjali. 1992. "Postpartum Contraception: Perspectives from Clients and Service Providers in Six Countries." *Final Report*. New York: Association for Voluntary Surgical Contraception.

Mauldin, W. P. and J. A. Ross. 1991. "Family planning programs: Efforts and results, 1982–89. *Studies in Family Planning* 22(6):350–367.

Population Council INOPAL II Program. 1992. "The Institutionalization of Postpartum Family Planning in Peru." *Final Report*. New York: The Population Council.

Ross, J. A., W. P. Mauldin, Steven R. Green, E. Romana Cooke. 1992. *Family Planning and Child Survival Programs as Assessed in 1991*. New York: The Population Council.

Rutenberg, N. and E. Landry. 1991. "Use and demand for sterilization: A comparison of recent findings from the demographic and health surveys." *Demographic and Health Surveys World Conference*, Columbia, Maryland: IRD/Macro International, Vol. 1:667–693.

Thapa, S., S. Kumar, J. Cushing, and K. Kennedy. 1992. "Contraceptive use among postpartum women: Recent patterns and programmatic implications." *International Family Planning Perspectives* 18(3):83–92.

Trussell, J., L. Grummer-Strawn, G. Rodriguez, and M. Vanlandingham. 1992. "Trends and differentials in breastfeeding behaviour: Evidence from the WFS and DHS." *Population Studies* 46(2):285–307.

Westoff, C. 1991. "Reproductive preferences: A comparative view." *Demographic and Health Surveys, Comparative Studies* No. 3. Columbia, MD: Institute for Resource Development/Macro Systems Inc.

Winikoff, B. and B. Mensch. 1991. "Rethinking postpartum family planning." *Studies in Family Planning* 22(5):294–307.

World Bank. 1992. *World Development Report 1992: Development and the Environment*. New York: Oxford University Press.

Zatuchni, G.I. 1970. "Overview of program: Two-year experience." In *Post-partum Family Planning: A Report on the International Program*. G.I. Zatuchni, ed. New York: McGraw-Hill.

Chapter 6

CHARGES AND PAYMENTS ASSOCIATED WITH PROVISION OF FAMILY PLANNING SERVICES

Governments must decide on appropriate charges for the family planning supplies and services they provide. These charges vary greatly across methods and countries, but programs usually subsidize family planning by providing services free. Some countries provide payments to contraceptive acceptors, motivators, and providers. Others charge for services. Price levels reflect competing goals: recovering costs to the program, maximizing the number of users, and simplifying the administrative tasks of service providers.

STRUCTURE OF PAYMENTS AND CHARGES

We distinguish among three categories: charges for services or methods, no charges, and payments to acceptors, providers, or motivators. *Table 1* classifies methods available from programs according to these price categories.

1. **Most developing countries provide most methods free of charge.**

   1.a. Of 59 developing countries for which information is available, 57 provide one or more methods free, while 35 provide all methods free. Only Singapore and Peru charge for all methods.

2. **Oral contraceptives and condoms are most likely to carry charges. Sterilization is least likely to carry a charge and most likely to carry a payment.**

   2.a. Of the 22 countries that make charges, all but seven charge for oral contraceptives and condoms. Only six countries charge for female sterilization, while two charge for male sterilization.

   2.b. As of 1989, six countries provided payments to sterilization acceptors; two provided payments to IUD acceptors.

3. **Pricing policies within countries are not always consistent across methods. These inconsistencies may reflect a desire to encourage the use of high continuation methods.**

   3.a. In 1989 Pakistan paid acceptors of (female) sterilization, but charged for reversible methods of contraception, such as pills and condoms.

   3.b. In the late 1980s India, Vietnam, and Bangladesh paid acceptors of IUDs and sterilization, but provided other methods free (Cleland and Mauldin, 1991).

   3.c. Panama and the Dominican Republic charged for sterilizations, but provided reversible methods free. Ghana charged for reversible methods, but provided sterilizations free (late 1980s).

TYPES OF PAYMENTS

Payments associated with contraceptive use or reproductive behavior can be classified according to the behavior for which the payment is made, who the recipient of the payment is, what the nature and the amount of the payment is, and when the payment is awarded.

4. **The most common type of payment to contraceptive adopters is a one-time cash award for sterilization or an IUD, as compensation for costs associated with adoption (such as lost work time and travel).**

   4.a. In the mid-1980s, the Indian program compensated sterilization and IUD acceptors for expenditures on drugs, meals, transportation to and from the clinic, and lost wages (US$9.00 for sterilization, $1.00 for IUDs) (Satia and Maru, 1986).

   4.b. Until recently sterilization acceptors in Bangladesh received the equivalent of about $5.50 (approximately one week's wages) and a sari or *lungi* to use as a clean surgical garment (Cleland and Mauldin, 1991).

   4.c. Between 1980 and 1989, Sri Lanka compensated sterilization acceptors for "actual and anticipated costs." The amount of the payment varied between the equivalent of $4.00 and $20.00 (De Silva et al., 1988).

   4.d. A pilot program in India demonstrated that small cash incentives attracted large numbers of

Table 1 Charges and payments to contraceptive acceptors, public sector, by country

Region	Charge acceptor fees Countries	Methods provided[a,b]	Neither charge nor pay acceptors Countries	Methods provided[a,c]	Region	Charge acceptor fees Countries	Methods provided[a,b]	Neither charge nor pay acceptors Countries	Methods provided[a,c]
Africa	Benin	I,O,In,C,S	Burkina Faso	All	Latin America/	Panama	I,O,St,S	Colombia	All
	Congo	I,O,In,C,S	Burundi	All	Caribbean	Peru	All	Costa Rica	All
	Ethiopia	I,O,S,D,St	Cameroon	All	(continued)	Puerto Rico	I,O,C,St,D,S	Dom. Rep.	I,O,C,S
	Ghana	I,O,In,C,St,S	Chad	All		Venezuela	I,St,S	Ecuador	All
	Guinea	I,O,In,C,S	Central African Rep.	All				El Salvador	All
	Lesotho	I,O,In,C,St,S	Ethiopia	In				Guyana	All
	Madagascar	I,O,In,C,St,D,S	Kenya	All				Haiti	All
	Nigeria	I,O,In,C,S	Mali	All				Honduras	All
	Zaire	I,O,In,C,St,S	Mauritania	All				Jamaica	All
			Mauritius	All				Mexico	All
			Mozambique	All				Nicaragua	All
			Niger	All				Panama	C
			Nigeria	St				Paraguay	All
			Rwanda	All				Trinidad & Tobago	All
			Sierra Leone	All				Venezuela	O,In
			Sudan	All	Asia	Hong Kong	I,O,In,C,St,D,S	Bangladesh	All
			Tanzania	All		Indonesia	N,St	China	All
			Togo	All		South Korea	O,C	Hong Kong	I,O,In,C,D,S
			Uganda	All		Malaysia	S,D,St(M),I,O,In,C	India	I,St
			Zambia	All		Pakistan	S,C,O	Indonesia	I,O,In,C
			Zimbabwe	All		Singapore	All	North Korea	All
Middle East	Lebanon	I,O,C,S	Morocco	All		Sri Lanka	O,C	South Korea	I,St,Ab
			Algeria	All		Taiwan	O,I,C	Malaysia	St(F)
			Tunisia	All				Mongolia	All
			Iran	All				Nepal	All
			Turkey	All				Pakistan	St,In,I
			Jordan	All				Philippines	All
			Syria	In,St,N				Sri Lanka	St,N,In,I
Latin America/								Taiwan	St
Caribbean	Dom. Rep.	St	Brazil	All				Thailand	All
	Guatemala	I,O,C,S	Chile	All				Vietnam	All

[a] Codes are: I = IUD; C = condoms; O = orals; In = injectables; St = sterilization (male or female); Ab = abortion; D = diaphragm; S = spermicides; N = NORPLANT®.
[b] The methods listed are those for which the countries charge.
[c] The methods listed are those for which the countries neither charge nor pay.

Notes: A few countries (listed below) provide payments to acceptors (usually only for sterilization or the IUD). Information is shown here as of 1989 (or 1987 in a few cases).

- Bangladesh: Sterilization ($5.42)
  IUD ($0.46)
- India: Sterilization ($0.62) (1987)
  IUD ($0.68) (1987)
- South Korea: Sterilization—Monetary subsidies to low-income sterilization acceptors for lost wages.
- Nepal: Sterilization ($3.68)
- Pakistan: Sterilization (female) ($1.00–$2.43)
- Sri Lanka: Sterilization ($13.87)
- Thailand: Sterilization ($4.44)
  IUD ($1.11)
- Vietnam: IUD ($1.00)
  Sterilization ($4.00)

Source: Ross et al., 1992.

women to clinics, where many of them accepted temporary methods. For some women, payments continued on a monthly basis after initial acceptance. Method continuation rates were unrelated to the duration for which payments were received (Stevens and Stevens, 1992).

5. Some programs pay motivators or, more commonly, providers of contraceptive services on a per-case basis. These payments may raise contraceptive prevalence by increasing the diffusion of information to potential acceptors and by encouraging health care providers to devote attention to family planning services.

5.a. In the Asian region, Indonesia, the Philippines, and Taiwan make per-case payments to service providers for oral pills; a few countries in other regions also do. A number of additional countries make per-case payments for IUD insertions and sterilizations (*Table 2*) (Ross et al., 1992).

5.b. India, Bangladesh, and Indonesia at different times have provided small payments to people who

Table 2 Public sector payments to providers[a] for contraceptive acceptance

Country	Female sterilization	Male sterilization	Intrauterine device	Oral contraceptives
Ethiopia	M	M	na	na
Lesotho	na	na	M	M
Sierra Leone	na	na	M	M
Lebanon	M,N	M,N	M,N	M,N
Colombia	M	M	na	na
Dom. Republic	M	M	M	O
El Salvador	O	O	O	O
Paraguay	M,O	na	na	na
Bangladesh	M,N	M,N	O	na
Indonesia	M	M	M,N	M,N
South Korea	M,O	M,O	M	na
Nepal	M,N,O	M,N,O	M,N	na
Pakistan	M,N,O	na	na	na
Philippines	O	O	O	O
Sri Lanka	M,N	M,N	na	na
Taiwan	O	O	O	M,N,O

[a] Provider codes are = M: medical doctors; N: nurses and/or midwives; O: others.
Notes: na = not applicable. Countries making no per-case payments: Angola, Botswana, Burkina Faso, Cameroon, Central African Republic, Chad, Congo, Ghana, Guinea, Madagascar, Mauritania, Mozambique, Nigeria, Rwanda, Senegal, Sudan, Tanzania, Togo, Uganda, Zaire, Zambia, Argentina, Chile, Costa Rica, Ecuador, Haiti, Jamaica, Mexico, Panama, Morocco, Tunisia, Turkey, Myanmar, China, Hong Kong, North Korea, Malaysia, Vietnam.
Source: Ross et al., 1992, Table 27.

motivate men and women to adopt contraception. The role of these motivators has varied from describing the steps involved in taking a method to accompanying sterilization acceptors to the clinic and providing support after the operation (Satia and Maru, 1986; Ancok, 1984).

5.c. Of 16 countries that make per-case payments, most pay medical personnel. Taiwan, the Philippines, and El Salvador pay non-medical workers. PROFAMILIA in Colombia provides per-case payments to workers in its community-based program; data from 1984 indicate an increase in sales due to these payments (Townsend, 1993).

6. **Some incentive schemes focus on communities. Designs vary, but the community typically receives rewards for attaining certain levels of contraceptive prevalence. Some rewards are a "public good," such as installation of a tube well. Other rewards may be passed on to individual contraceptors within the community.**

6.a. In a rural area of the Philippines, one bank granted loans at an interest rate of 10 percent (rather than 12 percent) to women who accepted contraception and did not get pregnant for one year (David, 1982). A similar scheme in Indonesia made funds for income-generating projects available to communities with high prevalence levels, but not to those with low levels. Women in high-prevalence communities who were family planning acceptors could borrow money from the funds at interest rates of only 1 or 2 percent (Ancok, 1984).

6.b. In Madhya Pradesh, India, village councils received money for development projects if they achieved sterilization targets. In Gujarat, village councils received one bag of cement for each vasectomy acceptor (Fincancioglu, 1982).

6.c. In one area of Thailand, village distributors of contraceptives purchased a water buffalo to rent to villagers. Rental rates were two times higher for noncontraceptors than for contraceptors (David and Viravaidya, 1986). In another area contraceptors could obtain larger loans than could noncontraceptors (Weeden et al., 1986).

6.d. Barnett (1987) lists a variety of community-level measures to reward the uptake of contraceptives in parts of Indonesia, Thailand, and India. However, clear evaluations of their effects have not been done.

7. **Some countries promote low fertility with non-cash incentives and disincentives, such as preferential access to health facilities and schools for small families.**

7.a. China provides advantages to only children and their parents, such as preference in housing allocation, supplements to monthly salaries, and priority in school admissions (Chen et al., 1982).

7.b. In Indonesia public servants do not receive any paid maternity leave after the first birth; rice allowances cover only a small number of children; and only three children can be deducted from taxes (Ancok, 1984).

7.c. Singapore has used a variety of incentives, first to reduce fertility and, after it fell to an alarmingly low level, to raise it among the better educated. Simultaneously, Singapore sought to discourage births among the less educated and poor by offering them substantial housing financing if they chose sterilization after the first or second child (mother below age 30), and also by raising the hospital delivery fee for third and later births (Singh et al., 1991).

7.d. In India some couples who have only two children and accept sterilization may receive a green card, which is meant to give them first priority in terms of loans, housing allotments, and medical facilities (Satia and Maru, 1986; Government of India, ca. 1986). However, in practice the card appears to have been little used.

7.e. Barnett's (1987) comprehensive compilation of the incentive and disincentive measures tried in various countries includes such examples as agricultural assistance to family planning acceptors, corporate tax exemptions for firms providing employees with family planning services, priority for government housing for contraceptors, and maternity leave for a limited number of children.

THE EFFECT OF PAYMENTS ON CONTRACEPTIVE USE

8. **Though the presence of compensation payments appears to be an important factor in clients' decisions to accept sterilization, most clients express a strong desire to limit family size as well.**

8.a. Evidence from detailed case studies of acceptors and surveys in Bangladesh indicates that the existence of compensation payments contributes to the decision to be sterilized (particularly for men) in a large number of cases (Cleland and Mauldin, 1991).

8.b. In focus-group discussions with sterilization acceptors in Bangladesh, all participants expressed a need to limit family size, regardless of whether they felt that the compensation payment had influenced their choice. Age and parity of acceptors did not vary seasonally or by level of payment, as one might expect if a financial motive were more important than a contraceptive motive (Cleland and Mauldin, 1991).

8.c. In Sri Lanka 60 percent of vasectomy acceptors were using contraceptives before their vasectomy. Increases in the payment did not change the percentage of acceptors saying they had wanted their wife's last pregnancy (De Silva et al., 1988).

9. **Payments or other rewards raise the prevalence levels of the methods for which rewards are offered.**

9.a. In South Asia almost two-thirds of acceptors use methods for which payments are made. In other regions (excluding China), only 12 percent of acceptors use the methods for which acceptance is compensated in South Asia (Mauldin and Sinding, 1992).

9.b. A community incentive program in Thailand resulted in much higher levels of contraceptive prevalence (all methods) and lower proportions of women pregnant in program villages where incentives were available than in matched control villages (see *Figure 1*). In the program villages prevalence rose from 46 percent to 76 percent, and the proportion pregnant fell from 10.9 percent to 5.4 percent. In the control villages prevalence rose from 51 percent to only 57 percent, and the proportion pregnant rose from 7.4 percent to 8.2 percent (Weeden et al., 1986).

9.c. In Sri Lanka monthly acceptance rates for sterilization varied directly with the level of the compensation payment. For example, the average number of monthly vasectomy acceptors was 1,030 when payments were the equivalent of $12.00 (January 1982–May 1983), but increased to 3,137 when payments increased to the equivalent of $20.00 (June 1983–December 1985) (Thapa et al., 1987).

9.d. In South Korea acceptance rates for sterilization increased by 67 percent for males and 53 percent for females in the months following the doubling of payments to acceptors, as compared to acceptance rates for the same months one year earlier. Increases in acceptance rates for IUDs, condoms, and pills were much smaller, at 31 percent, 7 percent, and 1 percent, respectively (Reditt, 1982).

10. **Where payments for method acceptance are available, the poor are more likely to adopt the compensated methods than are the rich.**

10.a. In Bangladesh, India, and Sri Lanka, sterilization acceptors receive compensation payments. In each of these countries, people of low economic status are more likely to choose sterilization than are people of higher economic status. In countries without compensation payments, there is no relationship between economic status and use of sterilization (Cleland and Mauldin, 1991).

10.b. In Sri Lanka levels of payment for acceptance of sterilization have fluctuated between the equivalent of $4.00 to $20.00. Higher levels of payments were accompanied by larger proportions of acceptors with incomes of less than about $40.00 per month (De Silva et al., 1988).

10.c. In a comparison of Bangladeshi women who had and had not undergone tubectomies, matched by village, number of living children, and desire for more children, the tubectomized women were worse off in a number of ways, including land and livestock ownership, household possessions, perceived inadequacy of income, and experience of a severe food shortage in the past five years (Cleland and Mauldin, 1991).

11. **Payments for sterilization acceptance probably**

Figure 1 Percentage of married women aged 15–44 in program and control villages practicing contraception (CPR) and percentage pregnant, Thailand, May 1983–May 1985

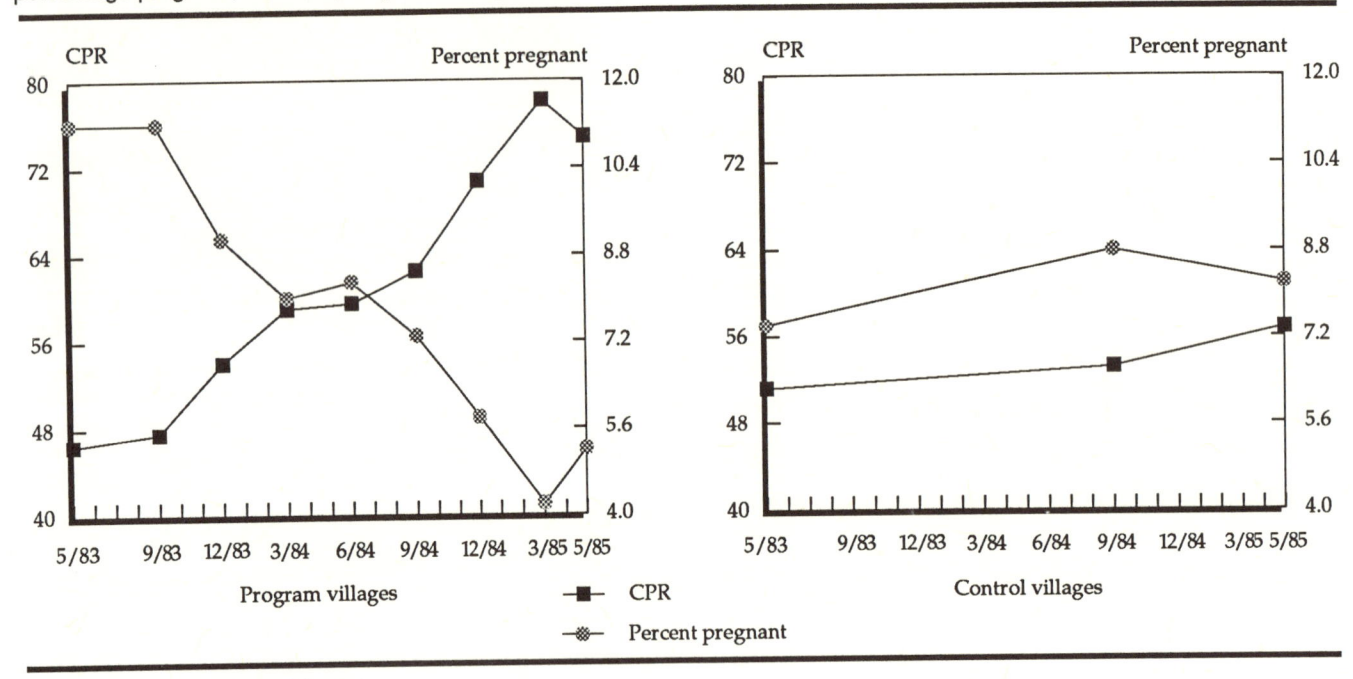

Source: Weeden et al., 1986, p. 12, Figure 1.
Reproduced with the permission of The Alan Guttmacher Institute from Donald Weeden, Anthony Bennett, Donald Lauro, and Mechai Viravaidya, "An Incentives Program to Increase Contraceptive Prevalence in Rural Thailand," *International Family Planning Perspectives*, Volume 12, No. 1, March 1986.

have a larger effect on the acceptance rates of men than of women.

11.a. The ratio of male to female acceptors of sterilization in Sri Lanka varied directly with the amount of the compensation payment (see *Figure 2*). In US$ equivalents, when the payment was $4.00 the ratio was approximately .35. When the payment was increased to $20.00 the ratio rose to 1.8. Later, when the payment was decreased to $8.00 the ratio fell back to approximately .25. Subsequently the payment was increased from $12.00 to $20.00 and the ratio increased again, from below .25 to about 1.2 (Thapa et al., 1987).

11.b. Similar evidence exists for Bangladesh. In 1983 payments to acceptors were increased from the equivalent of $4.00 to $7.00. The number of vasectomy acceptors more than doubled, while the number of tubectomy acceptors rose only 1.2 times (Cleland and Mauldin, 1991).

12. Payments to motivators are associated with increased use of methods for which the payments are offered.

12.a. Between April and June 1987, 99 percent of female and 84 percent of male sterilization acceptances in Bangladesh were associated with a third party. For men, 43 percent of these motivators were self-employed agents (rather than family planning field workers); for women, 25 percent of motivators were self-employed agents (Cleland and Mauldin, 1991).

12.b. In the mid-60s, the Tamil Nadu government paid the highest per-case fees to motivators of any Indian state. Correspondingly, acceptance rates for vasectomy in Tamil Nadu were over three times higher than in any other Indian state (Rogers, 1971).

12.c. In a 1970 experiment with rewards of powdered milk in Ghana, contraceptive acceptance levels were 1.6 times higher when both clients and motivators were milk recipients than when only the clients were, and three times higher than when neither was (Perkin, 1970).

THE EFFECT OF CHARGES ON CONTRACEPTIVE USE

Charging users for contraceptive supplies has advantages and disadvantages, both to the user and to the family planning program. If charges for services are reinvested in clinics, equipment, or more staff, charges may increase the efficiency with which services are supplied, reducing users' costs of travelling to clinics and waiting for appointments. A charge for contraceptives also implies

Figure 2 Ratio of male to female sterilization acceptors, Sri Lanka

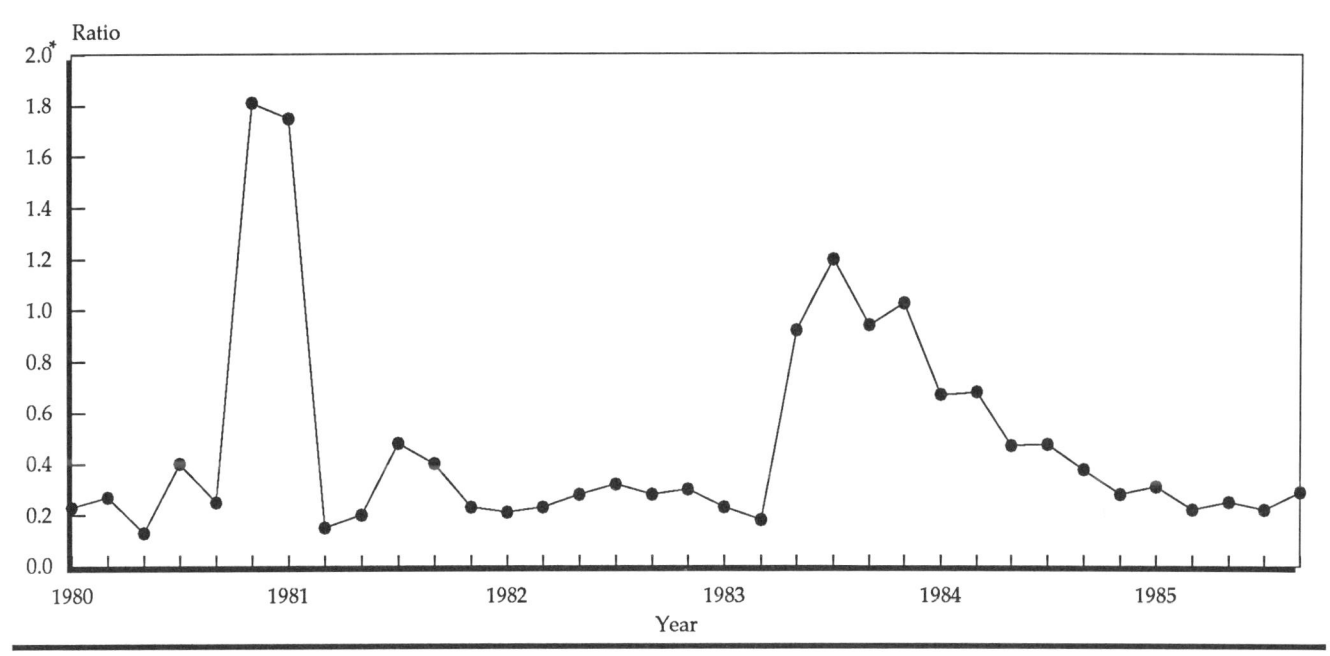

*Read: Two males for each female
Source: Thapa et al., 1987.

that the user is receiving something of value; moreover, potential acceptors may question the motives of agencies that provide products free. On the other hand, large volumes of small transactions are difficult administratively, and in economies with low levels of monetization, users may have a hard time finding cash for contraceptive supplies. One review (Lewis, 1986) of numerous studies concerning price elasticity in contraceptive use concludes that demand differs little between free services and moderately priced ones, and that modest rises in price have little effect on contraceptive use. Still, *reductions* in prices have considerably increased use.

13. **When prices are lowered, demand usually rises and clients may continue use of resupply methods longer.**

    13.a. In Taiwan a reduction in the price of oral contraceptives from the equivalent of $.25 to $.025 was accompanied by an increase of 2,500 to 6,000 cycles purchased per month (Cernada, 1982).

    13.b. In the fourth quarter of 1976 Thailand abolished charges for pills. The number of new users rose dramatically, from 81,000 to 125,000 by mid-1977. The number of new users of other methods increased by much less. The increase in pill use seemed not to be the result of women switching from other methods or sources (Knodel et al., 1984), although in some areas private sources of contraceptives that continued to charge fees lost business (Baldwin, 1978).

    13.c. Continuation rates for pills in Thailand were slightly higher for women who received the pill free than for women who paid (Knodel et al., 1984).

    13.d. In Turkey the Ankara Maternity Hospital provided free pills to clients, but due to a supply shortage began providing only prescriptions, which clients had to have filled at some expense. Continuation of use as of six months fell from 53 percent to 19 percent.

14. **Other evidence suggests that demand for contraceptives that cost only a small amount may not differ appreciably from demand for contraceptives that are free.**

    14.a. In Taiwan pills were offered at three different prices in three different areas: free, the equivalent of $.13, and the equivalent of $.25. The numbers of new acceptors were similar in the areas where pills were free or offered at $.13, but were only half as large in areas where $.25 was charged (Cernada, 1982).

    14.b. A pill distribution scheme in Egypt sent visitors to women's homes to offer four cycles of pills free. Women in one area were told they could visit a nearby clinic to receive additional free supplies. Women in another area were told they could visit a nearby clinic to purchase more supplies at $.05 per cycle. In both areas, prevalence rose from 19 percent to 27 percent over the nine-month study period (Gadalla et al., 1980).

14.c. In a Philippine study, women were more likely to choose methods for which a small price was charged than to choose those that were free, although beyond a certain threshold, the price discouraged selection of the method (Schwartz et al., 1989).

14.d. In Jamaica and Thailand the decision whether to purchase contraceptives or obtain them free was not affected by the price of the selected method (within a low range). Instead, a woman's age and occupation were more important; women of older age and higher status tended to purchase (Schwartz et al., 1989).

15. **Use of the more effective contraceptive methods may be less sensitive to price than is use of less effective methods. Price differentials favoring more effective methods may encourage women to choose these methods.**

15.a. In interviews in the Philippines and Thailand, suppositional increases in the price of condoms greatly lowered the predicted probability of use: the likelihood of choosing condoms was predicted to decrease by 45 percent, and 28 percent, respectively, for an increase of one standard deviation in price. However, percentage changes in the probability of choosing injectables, pills, and IUDs were much smaller, all below 7 percent. An increase in the price of sterilization in Thailand would decrease the probability of selecting sterilization by only 1.2 percent (Schwartz et al., 1989).

15.b. In two Thai provinces experimental price changes were introduced that raised the price of pills relative to injectables; these were followed by shifts from pills to injectables (Myers et al., 1991).

16. **When women are questioned about barriers to contraceptive use, very few mention cost as an issue. A partial exception occurs in Latin America, where some women are unable to obtain a tubectomy because of the expense.**

16.a. Participants in focus groups in Mexico almost never mentioned cost as a criterion for choosing one method over another, although cost appeared to affect the decision of where to obtain a method (Folch-Lyon et al., 1981).

16.b. The recent round of Demographic and Health Surveys asked women who had discontinued a method in the past five years why they had stopped using the method. Cost was rarely cited as the problem. The proportion of women who discontinued because of expense exceeded 5 percent only for injectables, and then in only four of over 20 countries (Bolivia, Guatemala, Thailand, and Indonesia).

16.c. In Brazil, Guatemala, and Honduras, women who were interested in sterilization but had not yet obtained it were asked why. Large proportions cited the cost of the procedure (Janowitz et al., 1985).

REFERENCES

Ancok, D. 1984. "Incentive and Disincentive Programs in Indonesian Family Planning." Yogyakarta, Indonesia: Population Studies Center, Gadja Mada University. Unpublished manuscript.

Baldwin, G. 1978. "The McCormick family planning program in Chiang Mai, Thailand." *Studies in Family Planning* 9(12):300–313.

Barnett, Patricia G. 1987. "Incentives for Family Planning?" Washington, DC: Population Crisis Committee.

Cernada, G. 1982. "How not to price oral contraceptives." In *Knowledge into Action: A Guide to Research Utilization*. Community Health Education Monographs. New York: Baywood Publishing Co., Inc.

Chen, P., X. Tian, and C. Tuan. 1982. "Eleven million Chinese opt for 'only child glory certificate.'" *People* 9(4):12–15.

Cleland, J. and W. P. Mauldin. 1991. "The promotion of family planning by financial payments: The case of Bangladesh." *Studies in Family Planning* 22(1):1–18.

David, H. 1982. "Incentives, reproductive behavior, and integrated community development in Asia." *Studies in Family Planning* 13(5):159–173.

David, H. and M. Viravaidya. 1986. "Community development and fertility management in rural Thailand." *International Family Planning Perspectives* 12(1):8–16.

De Silva, V., S. Thapa, L.R. Wilkens, M.G. Farr, K. Jayasinghe, and J.E. McMahan. 1988. "Compensatory payments and vasectomy acceptance in urban Sri Lanka." *Journal of Biosocial Science* 20(2):143–156.

Fincancioglu, N. 1982. "Carrots and sticks." *People* 9(4):3–10.

Folch-Lyon, E., L. DelaMacorra, and S. Schearer. 1981. "Focus group and survey research on family planning in Mexico." *Studies in Family Planning* 12(12):409–432.

Gadalla, S., N. Nosseir, and D. Gillespie. 1980. "Household distribution of contraceptives in rural Egypt." *Studies in Family Planning* 11(3):105–113.

Government of India. ca. 1986. "Revised strategy for national family welfare programme. A summary." New Delhi: Department of Family Welfare, Ministry of Health and Family Welfare.

Janowitz, B., J. Nunez, D. Covington, and C. Colven. 1985. "Why women don't get sterilized: A follow-up of women in Honduras." *Studies in Family Planning* 16(2):106–112.

Knodel, H., T. Bennett, and S. Panyadilok. 1984. "Do free pills make a difference? Thailand's experience." *International Family Planning Perspectives* 10(3):93–97.

Lewis, M.A. 1986. "Do contraceptive prices affect demand?" *Studies in Family Planning* 17(3):126–135.

Mauldin, W.P., and S.W. Sinding. 1992. "Review of existing family planning policies and programmes: Lessons learned." In *Family Planning, Health, and Family Wellbeing: Proceedings of the Expert Group Meeting*, Bangalore, India, 26–30 October. United Nations, forthcoming.

Myers, C.N., T. Ashakul, and S. Wattanalee. 1991. "Contraceptive repricing experimentation in Supanburi, Nakhon Sawan, Nakhon Sri Thammarat, and Surin." Unpublished manuscript.

Perkin, G.W. 1970. "Nonmonetary commodity incentives in family planning programs: A preliminary trial." *Studies in Family Planning* 1(57):12–15.

Reditt, J. 1982. "Incentives bring results." *People* 9(4):6–8.

Rogers, E.M. 1971. "Incentives in the diffusion of family planning innovations." *Studies in Family Planning* 2(12):241–248.

Ross, J. 1990 "Family planning pilot projects." In *Population Growth and Reproduction in Sub-Saharan Africa*. G. Ascadi, G. Johnson-Ascadi, and R. Bulatao, eds. Washington, DC: The World Bank.

Ross, J., W. Mauldin, S. Green, and E. Cooke. 1992. *Family Planning And Child Survival Programs As Assessed In 1991*. New York: The Population Council.

Satia, J.K. and R. Maru. 1986. "Incentives and disincentives in the Indian Family Welfare Program." *Studies in Family Planning* 17(3):136–145.

Schwartz, J., J. Akin, D. Guilkey, and V. Paqueo. 1989. "The effect of contraceptive prices on method choice in the Philippines, Jamaica, and Thailand." In *Choosing a Contraceptive: Method Choice in Asia and the United States*. R.A. Bulatao, J.A. Palmore, and S.E. Ward, eds. Boulder: Westview.

Singh, D., Y.F. Fong, and S.S. Ratnam. 1991. "A reversal of fertility trends in Singapore." *Journal of Biosocial Science* 23(1):73–78.

Stevens, J. and C. Stevens. 1992. "Introductory small cash incentives to promote child spacing in India." *Studies in Family Planning* 23(3):171–189.

Thapa, S., D. Abeywickrema, and L. Wilkens. 1987. "Effects of compensatory payments on vasectomy in urban Sri Lanka: A comparison of two economic groups." *Studies in Family Planning* 18(6):352–360.

Townsend, John. 1993. Personal communication.

Weeden, D., A. Bennett, D. Lauro, and M. Viravaidya. 1986. "An incentives program to increase contraceptive prevalence in rural Thailand." *International Family Planning Perspectives* 12(1):11–16.

Chapter 7

CONTRACEPTIVE CONTINUATION AND EFFECTIVENESS

Whatever the adoption rate for contraception, better continuation raises prevalence quite sharply. Further, as prevalence rises, method effectiveness increasingly determines the fertility level, since the failure rate involved applies to larger numbers of couples.

Information on continuation and effectiveness comes from three basic sources: clinic data, program information, and household surveys. The first has provided precise estimates of continuation and failure rates for individual contraceptive methods; the second has produced rates that reflect more general field conditions; and the third has afforded a picture of behavior in the general population.[1]

Some continuation and failure rates are *aggregated*, which involves merging data across all durations of use and converting them to an artificial annual measure. Others derive from life-table techniques, based on a separate rate for each month of use, with cumulation of monthly continuation rates to estimate the proportion of original acceptors still contracepting after each period of time. The life-table failure rate estimates the proportion of original acceptors who would have experienced a contraceptive failure by each interval of time. Most rates given below are from life-table estimates and pertain chiefly to developing countries. Because studies vary greatly in their definitions and procedures, results are presented by method and source of information. For other reviews of methodology and detailed results, see Trussell and Kost (1987), Jejeebhoy (1989), and Bongaarts and Rodriguez (1991).

The subject of continuation takes on particular importance regarding overall prevalence of use (see Chapter 1). As *Figure 1* illustrates, prevalence is much more sensitive to the annual continuation rate than it is to the acceptance rate. Prevalence can rise to 50 percent of the population even though the acceptance rate is as low as 5 percent, providing the annual continuation rate among users is 90 percent (Jain, 1989; cited in Bruce and Jain, 1991). The continuation rate varies greatly among contraceptive methods, but a variety of method choices helps couples initiate contraception earlier and find alternative protection when their method becomes unsatisfactory.

CONTRACEPTIVE CONTINUATION RATES

1. **Contraceptive continuation varies across methods. Variation also exists within each method: continuation for the IUD is typically longer than that for the pill, which, in turn, exceeds that for the condom. Injectable continuation rates appear to vary substantially. Information to date gives high continuation for the NORPLANT® method. Rates for all methods also differ depending upon the data source (clinic, program, survey).**

Estimates below, unless otherwise cited, come from a general review of the literature (Frankenberg and Ross, 1992).

Oral Contraceptives

1.a. Most 12-month continuation rates for oral contraceptives fall between 40 percent and 60 percent. Regardless of the type of data (clinic, program, or survey), the median is 45–50 percent. The range of estimates from program data (23–72 percent from 13 studies) is wider than that from clinic data (40–64 percent from seven studies). An extensive review of early experience found a wide range of continuation rates, from 25 percent to 80 percent for all types of data, which agrees with the outside limits of ranges above (Mason, 1970).

IUDs

1.b. For IUDs 12-month continuation rates typically fall between 70 percent and 85 percent, above those for the pill, even after taking account of age and family size. The median from program data (74 percent from 13 studies) is considerably lower than the median from clinic data (83 percent from 15 studies). Program estimates range from 48 percent to 92 percent, while clinic estimates range from 68 percent to 90 percent.

Injectables

1.c. Twelve-month continuation rates for injectables vary substantially, but are generally lower for clinic data than for program data. Estimates from clinic data range from 22 percent to 63 percent, with a median of around 38 percent (based on six studies). Estimates from program data range from 50 percent to 75 percent, with a median of 60 percent (based on six studies).

Figure 1 Contraceptive prevalence rate resulting from various combinations of annual acceptance and continuation rates per 100 married women of reproductive age (MWRA)

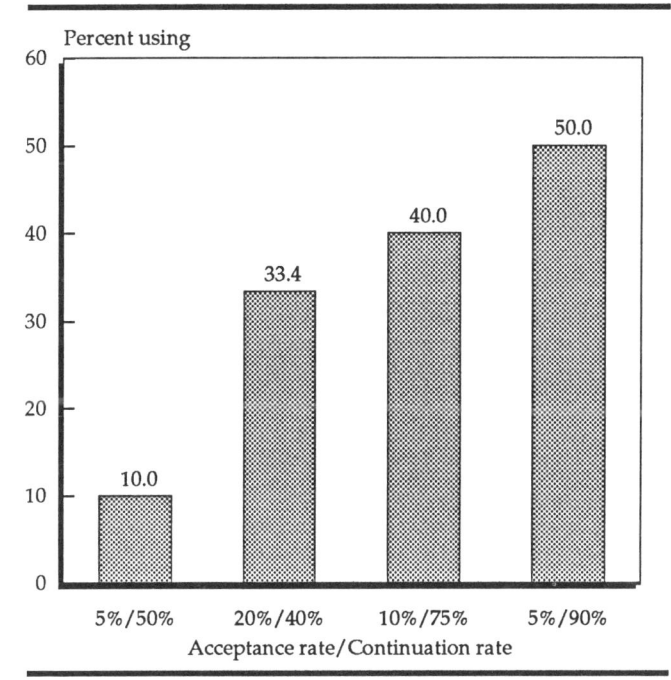

Percent using

Acceptance rate/Continuation rate	Percent
5%/50%	10.0
20%/40%	33.4
10%/75%	40.0
5%/90%	50.0

Source: Bruce and Jain, 1991.

NORPLANT®

1.d. Estimates of one-year continuation rates for NORPLANT®, all from clinic data, range from 80 percent in Scandinavia to 94 percent in China and 95 percent in Chile. Two-year continuation rates are 67 percent or higher (Sivin, 1988).

Condoms

1.e. The few studies available suggest that 12-month continuation rates for condoms are no higher than 45 percent.

Periodic Abstinence

1.f. Clinic, survey, and program data on continuation of periodic abstinence suggest that 38 percent to 42 percent of initial acceptors are continuing method use at 12 months. Two studies put the rate higher, at about 62 percent.

2. In longer-term data,[2] women appear to be protected from pregnancy more effectively than extrapolation of 12-month, first-segment, or first-method rates would imply.

The following evidence is from a long-term follow-up of IUD acceptors in Taichung, Taiwan (Moots and Chen, 1973). (Although the data are from the early history of family planning programs, they illustrate important points.)

2.a. Termination rates projected for years eight and nine of the study, from data on IUD termination rates in previous years, underestimated the extent to which women would continue use.

2.b. At the beginning of the study, 81 percent of the IUD acceptors had never previously used a contraceptive method, but during the study period the percentage using some effective method never fell below 65 percent.

2.c. The percentage of IUD acceptors still using their first IUD was 30 percent at 54 months of use and 19 percent at 104 months. However, when reinsertions of IUDs were considered, over 50 percent of the women were still using an IUD 90 months into the study.

CONTRACEPTIVE FAILURE RATES

Failure rates are usually given only for the early years of use, but these can be deceptive for the longer term (*Figure 2*). The effectiveness level must be very high to reduce the 10 year risk of failure below 1 percent.

3. As with continuation, failure rates vary widely by method, within method, and by source of information. However, they are nearly zero for both male and female sterilization, low for injectables and NORPLANT®, very low for the newer, improved IUDs, and low for the pill when properly used (though higher in practice). Failure rates are much higher for condoms and periodic abstinence.

Sterilization

3.a. Failure rates in US data for both male and female sterilization are extremely low, estimated at 0.4 and 0.15 over one year per 100 users for females and males, respectively (Trussell and Kost, 1987). In developing country data most 12 month life-table failure rates range from 0.2 to 0.6 (Ross et al., 1985).

Oral Contraceptives

3.b. Estimates of one-year failure rates for pills hover around 1 percent, according to clinic data. The me-

Figure 2 Relation of contraceptive failure to effectiveness levels

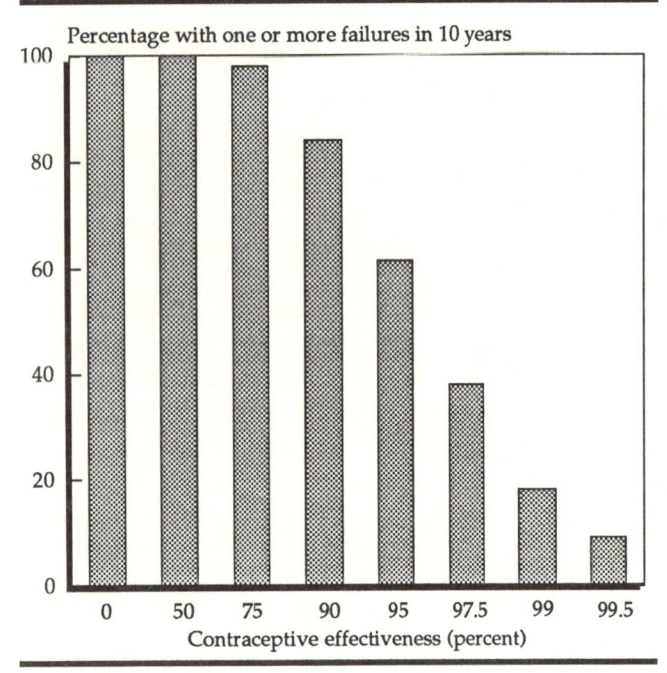

[Bar chart: Percentage with one or more failures in 10 years vs Contraceptive effectiveness (percent). Bars at effectiveness levels 0, 50, 75, 90, 95, 97.5, 99, 99.5 showing approximately 100, 100, 98, 84, 62, 38, 18, 9 percent respectively.]

Source: Ross et al., 1989, p. 39.

dian failure rates from program and survey data are 5 percent (nine studies) and 6.4 percent (17 studies), respectively. Estimates from survey data range from 2.7 percent to 14 percent, while estimates from program data range widely, from zero to 26 percent.

IUDs

3.c. Failure rates of IUDs are low, but vary by technological features of the device. Nonmedicated devices and the earliest copper IUDs have failure rates above 2 per 100 woman-years of use. The most recent and widely used copper IUDs have failure rates significantly below that. As the copper surface area of the IUD increases from 200 to 350 mm² or more, pregnancy rates decrease from 2.1 per 100 woman-years to 0.4 per 100 woman-years. IUDs releasing at least 20 mcg/day of levonorgestrel also have very low failure rates. IUDs releasing progesterone have significantly higher failure rates than the best copper IUDs. (Estimates are from multicenter randomized trials of IUDs conducted between 1970 and 1990, encompassing more than 50,000 woman-years of experience) (Sivin and Schmidt, 1987; Sivin, 1991).

Injectables

3.d. Most data for failure rates of injectables are from clinical trials; 12-month rates are zero to 1 percent.

NORPLANT®

3.e. First-year Pearl pregnancy rates for NORPLANT® capsules are 0.2 per 100 woman-years (based on over 12,000 woman-years of use in 11 countries), and 0.2 in the second year (9 countries, 5,800 woman-years of use). Excluding China both rates were 0.3 (Sivin, 1988).

Condoms

3.f. Program estimates of 12-month failure rates for condoms, chiefly from developed countries, vary from 10 percent to 24 percent. One clinic estimate from the Caribbean puts the failure rate at 4 percent (Bailey and Keller, 1982), but few studies of condom failure in developing countries are available. Condom breakage can cause failure; breakage rates in actual practice may range from 7–13 percent (prospective studies reported by Russell-Brown et al., 1992). However, retrospective reports by 282 US respondents gave an average of one break per 161 uses of condoms (Hatcher et al., 1988).

Periodic Abstinence

3.g. Failure rates for periodic abstinence from Demographic and Health Survey data (14 developing countries) range from 8.2 percent to 38.4 percent, around a median of 19.9 percent (Moreno and Goldman, 1991). Program data from the Philippines put failure rates at 14–20 percent (Laing, 1984a, 1984b, 1986).

CORRELATES OF CONTINUATION: SIDE EFFECTS, MEDICAL REASONS, AND FAILURES

4. For IUDs, NORPLANT®, and injectables, side effects (particularly menstrual irregularities) are by far the most important reasons for discontinuation.

4.a. For the IUD, side effects caused most terminations in a multicenter World Health Organization study and in studies of different types of IUDs in seven countries. In six of the studies menstrual disturbances and pain ranked first among reasons for IUD discontinuation. In another five studies side effects were the second most important reason for discontinuation, while "other medical reasons" were also important (Bhatia and Kim, 1984; Shaaban et al., 1983; World Health Organization, 1990; Somboonsuk et al., 1978).

4.b. A study of IUD acceptors in Mexico City found that women who unexpectedly experience increases in menstrual blood loss are more likely to discontinue IUD use than are other women (Zetina-Lozano, 1983).

4.c. For injectable contraceptives, side effects or medical reasons are the first or second most important reason for discontinuation in Thailand, Bangladesh, Mexico, Egypt, and Pakistan. In Mexico and Pakistan menstrual disturbances and "other medical reasons" rank no lower than third among reasons for discontinuation (Somboonsuk et al., 1978; Meade et al., 1984; Kazi et al., 1985; Narkavonnakit et al., 1982; Salem et al., 1988).

4.d. For NORPLANT®, in Indonesia, Egypt, Chile, China, India, and Thailand, women are most at risk of terminating use because of menstrual problems or pain. "Other medical reasons" are important in all countries except Thailand (Lubis et al., 1983; Shabaan, 1983; Salah et al., 1987; Gu et al., 1988; Indian Council of Medical Research., 1988; Somboonsuk et al., 1978; Marangoni et al., 1983).

4.e. For the IUD and NORPLANT®, short-term and long-term experience tend to differ. Terminations in the first few years are due more to medical reasons, principally menstrual problems; thereafter, personal reasons, especially planning a pregnancy, become more important (Sivin, 1993).

5. **Among pill users, side effects and medical reasons explain a substantial portion of discontinuations.**

    5.a. Side effects or medical reasons for pill discontinuation ranked first among women in Indonesia, Thailand, and Bangladesh (Teachman et al.,1980; Somboonsuk et al., 1978; Bhatia and Kim, 1984).

    5.b. In Sri Lanka, among pill users who switched to traditional methods, side effects were cited as the reason for doing so three times more often than the second most important reason, desire for more children (Kane et al., 1988).

    5.c. In pre-1970 studies, side effects accounted for a large portion of pill discontinuation (Mauldin et al., 1967). Kreager (1977) reached a similar conclusion in an extensive review of discontinuation in developing countries.

    5.d. A survey of perceptions of the pill's safety that was conducted in eight developing countries found that over 40 percent of women viewed the pill as being more physically dangerous than childbearing (Grubb, 1987).

    5.e. Health concerns were not included as a reason for pill discontinuation in Peru or the Philippines. In both of these countries, however, discontinuation for the purpose of immediately switching methods was common (Kost, 1990; Choe and Zablan, 1991).

6. **Failure is an important reason for discontinuation of pills, condoms, and traditional methods.**

    6.a. Accidental pregnancy is a major reason for termination of pill use in Peru, the Philippines, and Bangladesh (Kost, 1990; Choe and Zablan, 1991; Bhatia and Kim, 1984). Accidental pregnancy was not, however, an important reason for discontinuation in early studies in Indonesia or Thailand (Teachman et al., 1980; Somboonsuk et al., 1978).

    6.b. Failure is an important factor in discontinuation of condom use in studies where data are available on reasons (Bangladesh, Indonesia, and the Philippines) (Bhatia and Kim, 1984; Teachman et al., 1980; Choe and Zablan, 1991).

    6.c. Many rhythm users in the Philippines and Peru discontinue the practice because of method failure (Kost, 1990; Choe and Zablan, 1991). In Bangladesh accidental pregnancy is a common cause of discontinuation among users of traditional methods (Bhatia and Kim, 1984).

Results from Demographic and Health Surveys

7. **For 10 developing countries DHS surveys indicate why women discontinued methods tried in the past five years.[3] The most common reasons given for discontinuation of pills and IUDs were desire for pregnancy and concern about side effects and health problems. Method failure and "other" reasons were substantially less important, but still accounted for an appreciable portion of discontinuation. Reasons rarely cited for stopping included inconvenience, partner's disapproval, poor access and availability, cost, and infrequent sex; however, these are the very reasons that can prevent starting a method in the first place.**

    7.a. For former users of oral contraceptives, health concerns and fears of side effects ranked first among reasons for discontinuation in six countries, while desire for additional children ranked second. In the remaining four countries the ranking of these two reasons was reversed. In each country the two reasons together accounted for more than 50 percent of pill discontinuations.

7.b. For IUD users health concerns accounted for the largest proportion of discontinuations in eight countries, while desire for another pregnancy ranked second. In the remaining two countries the ranking of the reasons was reversed. Health concerns and desire for more children, taken together, explained over 50 percent of IUD discontinuations in each country.

7.c. Method failure always ranked third or fourth in importance among reasons for discontinuation, for both pills and IUDs.

7.d. Partner disapproval and method inconvenience were never cited as the reason for discontinuation by more than 5 percent of respondents. Infrequent sex and issues of access, availability, or cost were mentioned only slightly more often.

7.e. In Thailand and Sri Lanka nearly 9 percent of women discontinued the IUD to switch to another method.

CORRELATES OF CONTINUATION: PERSONAL CHARACTERISTICS

Note: Most studies examine only bivariate relationships, rather than several factors together in a multivariate model, and many group all contraceptive methods together.

8. **Typically, older women have higher rates of contraceptive continuation than do younger women.**

    8.a. Average annual continuation rates in the Philippines (1980) increased by age from 43 percent (ages 20–24) to 83 percent (ages 45–49) (Laing, 1985).

    8.b. In Indonesia (all methods combined) early 12-month continuation rates ranged from 41 percent for women aged 25 and under to 64 percent for women aged 36 to 49 (Teachman et al., 1980).

    8.c. Among injectable acceptors in Thailand, continuation rates increased until age 40, then declined (Narkavonnakit et al., 1982).

    8.d. In Matlab, Bangladesh, the probability of continuation as of five years after adoption (all methods combined) was significantly higher for older women than for younger women (Rahman et al., 1990).

    8.e. Early reviews showed IUD continuation rates to rise regularly with age in carefully conducted studies in Taichung (Potter et al., 1967), in Taiwan as a whole (Chow et al., 1967), and in the United States (Tietze, 1967). Age patterns were irregular in two early studies from Thailand and India (Mauldin et al., 1967). Pill continuation showed a mixed age pattern; if anything it declined among older women (aged 35 or more), perhaps because users found it easy to stop as they experienced declining fecundity or menopause (Jones and Mauldin, 1967; Kraeger, 1977).

9. **The effect of parity on contraceptive continuation is somewhat mixed, but the relationship is generally positive.**

    9.a. In the Dominican Republic a multivariate analysis showed contraceptive continuation to increase significantly with parity (Porter, 1984). Similar results were obtained in a bivariate analysis of Indonesian data, where women with two or fewer children had a 12-month continuation rate of 39 percent, while women with more than two children had rates of over 52 percent (Teachman et al., 1980).

    9.b. In Thailand 24-month continuation rates for users of the injectable increased with parity, from 33 percent for women with two or fewer children to 47 percent for women with more than two (Narkavonnakit et al., 1982).

    9.c. In Bangladesh the number of children ever born was not a significant predictor of continuation after controlling for sex composition of the family; however, sex composition was a good predictor (Rahman et al., 1990) (see below).

    9.d. Among users of the rhythm method in the Philippines, continuation rates in an early study decreased with parity (Phillips, 1978).

    9.e. Early reviews showed that IUD continuation rates rose regularly with parity in the studies cited above (for age trends) for Taichung, Taiwan, and the United States. However, for the pill, continuation patterns by parity were mixed and inconclusive (Jones and Mauldin, 1967).

10. **In countries where son preference is strong, sex composition of the family affects contraceptive continuation.**

    10.a. In Menoufia, Egypt, women with more sons were more likely to accept oral contraception and still be using it as of nine months than were women with fewer sons, controlling for parity (Gadalla et al., 1985).

10.b. In Matlab, Bangladesh, bivariate analysis showed a strong relationship between family sex composition and contraceptive continuation. Among four- and five-child families, no women lacking sons were continuing contraceptive use at 60 months, while for women with at least one son, the rates were 46 percent and 50 percent, respectively (Rahman et al., 1990).

10.c. In Matlab the strength of the relationship remained when socioeconomic controls were introduced. The risk of discontinuation was 44 percent lower for women with one or more sons than for women with no sons. (For women with one or more daughters the risk was 33 percent lower than for women with no daughters, suggesting that parents want at least one daughter) (Rahman et al., 1990).

11. **Education does not appear to have a strong effect on contraceptive continuation.**

    11.a. Female education was not a significant determinant of continuation in the Dominican Republic, the Philippines, South Korea, Trinidad and Tobago, or Matlab, Bangladesh (Porter, 1984; Park and Kong, 1987; Abdulah, 1988, 1990; Phillips, 1978; Rahman et al., 1990).

    11.b. Early studies of IUD use in Turkey found no relationship between education or literacy and continuation (Ross et al., 1972).

    11.c. In Matlab, Bangladesh, however, women living in households headed by someone with a primary school education had significantly higher probabilities of continuation than did women living in other households (Rahman et al., 1990).

12. **Desire for more children affects continuation.**

    12.a. In the Philippines women who did not want more children had continuation rates 11 percentage points higher than those of women who desired additional children (73 percent vs. 62 percent, respectively) (Laing, 1985).

    12.b. In Thailand injectable users who did not want any more children had continuation rates 50 percent higher than those who did want more children (Narkavonnakit et al., 1982).

CORRELATES OF FAILURE
Results from Demographic and Health Surveys

Differentials in contraceptive failure in 15 developing countries are available from Demographic and Health Survey data (Moreno, 1991). Across *countries*, median failure rates are compared, and across *individuals*, failure risks are compared (by proportional hazards techniques).

13. *By method*: **Across countries life-table failure rates are more than two times higher for barrier and traditional methods than for effective modern methods. The pattern remains after controlling for education and residence.**

    13.a. Across the 15 countries the median 12-month failure rate for effective methods (pill, IUD, injectable, and implant) was only 5.6 percent, while for traditional methods (rhythm and withdrawal) and barrier methods (condoms and vaginal methods), the median failure rates were 18.4 percent and 16.3 percent, respectively. This ordering remains within categories of residence and education.

    13.b. Across individuals the type of contraceptive method was the best predictor of failure (single-factor analyses).

14. *By age and parity*: **Across countries age and parity were generally the second most important predictors of failure after method. Other, non-DHS evidence shows that age affects failure rates for IUDs.**

    14.a. Generally, younger women have higher failure rates than older women. In one Scandinavian trial 35 year-olds had only 35 percent of the risk of failure of 25 year-olds (Allonen et al., 1984). Older women may be more likely to be sterile or may have intercourse less frequently than younger women (Sivin and Schmidt, 1987).

15. *By residence and education*: **Generally, urban and better educated women have lower failure rates, although results are variable.**

    15.a. Across countries, for effective and barrier methods, failure rates are slightly lower in urban than in rural areas, but the differences are not statistically significant. For traditional methods the median failure rate is 22 percent in urban areas, but only 15 percent in rural areas. Regardless of method type, estimates for rural areas are more wide-ranging than for urban areas.

    15.b. Across individuals the relationship between

residence and risk of failure was statistically significant in only six of the 15 countries: Bolivia, Ecuador, Colombia, Peru, Sri Lanka, and Tunisia. Where residence was important, rural women had failure rates up to twice those of urban women. In Colombia and Sri Lanka residence effects were not significant.

15.c. Across countries failure rates do not vary clearly by educational level (less than secondary, secondary, and higher than secondary). The range of failure rates across countries is smallest for the category of secondary education.

15.d. Across individuals education effects on the risk of failure were statistically significant in the same six countries as in 15.b. (for residence), as well as in Thailand and the Dominican Republic. Where education was important, women with at least a secondary level of education failed less frequently than did their less-educated counterparts.

16. *By duration of use*: **In some data sets failure rates change depending upon which year of use is involved.**

16.a. In several countries duration of use was as important as age and parity in affecting failure. However, the relationship between duration of use and failure varies substantially from country to country, even after controlling for method, age, and parity. In over half of the 15 countries duration of use was not related to the risk of failure at a statistically significant level. In seven countries the risk of failure declined as duration of use increased, suggesting that women most likely to experience a failure do so soon after adopting a method, leaving a residue of more successful contraceptors.

16.b. In five countries the risk of failure is greatest between six and 11 months of use. The risk possibly peaks at this point rather than at 0–5 months because women who adopt contraception shortly after a birth are protected from an early conception by postpartum infecundability.

16.c. In the United States (non-DHS data), failure rates for reversible contraceptives are lower in the fourth year of use than in the third year of use, and are lower in the third year of use than in the last quarter of the second year of use. This pattern holds for pills, IUDs, condoms, rhythm, and withdrawal (Westoff, 1988).

17. **After an accidental pregnancy many women return to the same method as before.**

17.a. In Peru 51 percent of rhythm users who failed resumed the rhythm method within 12 months after the pregnancy ended. For pill users experiencing an accidental pregnancy, the figure was 42 percent (Kost, 1990).

17.b. In Trinidad and Tobago almost all women who became pregnant while using a barrier method or a traditional method readopted that method after the pregnancy. About two-thirds of women who experienced a method failure with the pill or IUD resumed use of the method (Abdulah, 1988, 1990).

17.c. In South Korea far more women who became pregnant while using the pill or condom returned to that method after the pregnancy than did women who discontinued the methods for other reasons (Park and Kong, 1987).

18. **Programs that offer a variety of method choices may encourage continued effective contraceptive use by providing reliable alternatives to couples dissatisfied with a current or recently discontinued method.**

18.a. Countries with strong family planning programs (see Chapter 2) tend to have low failure rates. Across 15 countries with DHS surveys the correlation between program strength and the failure rate (all methods) is –0.75, or –0.68 excluding sterilization. Two Asian countries with especially strong programs (Thailand and Indonesia) and one in Latin America (Mexico) have the lowest failure rates by a substantial margin (Moreno and Goldman, 1991).

18.b. In Matlab, Bangladesh, fieldworkers are trained to encourage dissatisfied users to adopt other methods. This strategy has improved overall persistence of use, as shown by a comparison of first-method and all-method continuation rates for different cohorts of adopters (Akbar et al., 1990).

18.c. In Surabaya, Indonesia, women who received their first choice of a contraceptive method were far more likely to continue use than were other women. For example, 98 percent of those who received the pill but wanted another method discontinued within a year, versus only 26 percent of women who chose the pill and received it (Pariani et al., 1987).

NOTES

1. Population-based retrospective data have four disadvantages. First, respondents sometimes provide inaccurate information on past contraceptive behavior. Second, if surveys collect information only on selected intervals of use (such as the most recent ones), esti-

mates of continuation and failure rates may be biased, depending on the analytic question. Third, many surveys do not collect data on pregnancies (including accidental pregnancies) that result in a miscarriage, which biases failure rates downward (Goldman et al., 1991). Finally, determining whether or not a birth was unplanned may be difficult. Inclusion of planned births in the estimation of failure rates can seriously bias results (Goldman et al., 1983).

2. Short-term rates pertain either to a particular segment of method use or a particular method used within a limited time interval. Once that segment or method is terminated or the time period ends, information on the woman's subsequent contraceptive use is not generally available.

3. Women were asked the main reason why they terminated the method used immediately prior to each birth (if any) that occurred within five years of the interview. Data on reasons for termination are available from Thailand, the Dominican Republic, Egypt, Bolivia, Colombia, Sri Lanka, Guatemala, Paraguay, Indonesia, and Trinidad and Tobago.

REFERENCES

Abdulah, N. 1988. "Variations according to background characteristics in method continuation and failure: The case of Trinidad and Tobago." Unpublished. (IESA/P/AC. 27/16).

———. 1990. "Selection, change, and discontinuation of contraceptive methods in Trinidad and Tobago." *Demographic and Health Surveys Further Analysis* No. 4. Columbia, Maryland: IRD/Macro International.

Akbar, J., J. Phillips, and M. Koenig. 1990. "Trends in contraceptive method mix, continuation rates, and failure rates in Matlab, Bangladesh: 1978–87." In *Measuring the Dynamics of Contraceptive Use*. New York: United Nations.

Allonen, H. et al. 1984. "Factors affecting the clinical performance of Nova T and Copper T 300." *Obstetrics and Gynecology* 64:524–529.

Bailey, J. and A. Keller. 1982. "Post-family planning acceptance experience in the Caribbean: St. Kitts-Nevis and St. Vincent." *Studies in Family Planning* 13(2):44–58.

Bhatia, S. and Y. Kim. 1984. "Oral contraception in Bangladesh." *Studies in Family Planning* 15(5):233–241.

Bongaarts, J. and G. Rodriguez. 1991. "A new method for estimating contraceptive failure rates." In *Measuring the Dynamics of Contraceptive Use*. New York: Department of International Economic and Social Affairs, United Nations (ST/ESA/SER.R.106).

Bruce, J. and A.K. Jain. 1991. "Improving the quality of care through operations research." In *Operations Research: Helping Family Planning Programs Work Better*. M. Seidman and M.C. Horn, eds. New York: Wiley-Liss.

Choe, M.K. and Z.C. Zablan. 1991. "Contraceptive use and discontinuation and failure rates in the Philippines: Estimates from the 1986 Contraceptive Prevalence Survey." In *Measuring the Dynamics of Contraceptive Use*. New York: Department of International Economic and Social Affairs, United Nations (ST/ESA/SER.R.106).

Chow, L.P., R. Freedman, R.G. Potter, and A.K. Jain. 1967. "Correlates of IUD termination in a mass family planning program: The first Taiwan follow-up survey." *Studies in Family Planning* 1(24):13–16.

Frankenberg, E. and J.A. Ross. 1992. "A review of contraceptive continuation rates in the developing world." Unpublished manuscript.

Gadalla, S., S. McCarthy, and O. Campbell. 1985. "How the number of living sons influences contraceptive use in Menoufia Governorate, Egypt." *Studies in Family Planning* 16(3):164–169.

Goldman, N., L. Moreno, C. Westoff, and B. Vaughan. 1991. "Estimates of contraceptive failure and discontinuation based on two methods of contraceptive data collection in Peru." In *Measuring the Dynamics of Contraceptive Use*. New York: Department of International Economic and Social Affairs, United Nations (ST/ESA/SER.R.106).

Goldman, N., A. Pebley, C. Westoff, and L. Paul. 1983. "Contraceptive failure rates in Latin America." *International Family Planning Perspectives* 9(2):50–57.

Grubb, G.S. 1987. "Women's perceptions of the safety of the pill: A survey in eight developing countries." *Journal of Biosocial Science* 19:313–321.

Gu, S.J., M.G. Du, D.Y. Yuan, L.D. Zhang, M.F. Xu, Y.L. Liu, S.H. Wang, S.L. Wu, P.Z. Wang, Y.L Gao, X. He, L.F. Qi, C.R. Chen, Y.P. Liu, P. Mo, and I. Sivin. 1988. "A two-year study of acceptability, side effects, and effectiveness of NORPLANT® and NORPLANT-2® implants in the People's Republic of China." *Contraception* 38(6):641–657.

Hatcher, R.A. et al. 1988. *Contraceptive Technology: 1988–1989. 14th revised edition*. New York: Irvington Publishers.

Indian Council of Medical Research. 1988. "Phase III-clinical trial with NORPLANT-2® (covered rods). Report of a 24-month study." *Contraception* 38(6): 659–673.

Jain, A.K. 1989. "Fertility reduction and the quality of family planning services." *Studies in Family Planning* 20(1):1–16.

Jejeebhoy, S. 1989. "Measuring the quality and duration of contraceptive use: An overview of new approaches." *Population Bulletin of the United Nations* 26:1–38. New York: United Nations.

Jones, G.W. and W.P. Mauldin. 1967. "Use of oral contraceptives: With special reference to developing countries." *Studies in Family Planning* 1(24):1–13.

Kane, T., K. Gaminaratne, and E. Stephen. 1988. "Contraceptive method-switching in Sri Lanka: Patterns and implications." *International Family Planning Perspectives* 14(2):68–75.

Kazi, A., S. Holck, and P. Diethelm. 1985. "Phase IV study of the injection Norigest in Pakistan." *Contraception* 32(4):395–403.

Kost, K. 1990. "Contraceptive discontinuation in Peru: Patterns and demographic implications." Ph.D. dissertation presented to the faculty of Princeton University. Krager, P. 1977. *Family planning dropouts reconsidered*. London: International Planned Parenthood Federation.

Krager, P. 1977. *Family Planning Dropouts Reconsidered*. London: International Planned Parenthood Federation.

Laing, J. 1984a. "Natural family planning in the Philippines." *Studies in Family Planning* 15(2):49–61.

———. 1984b. "Research on natural family planning in the Philippines." In *Natural Family Planning: Development of National Programs*. C.A. Lanctot, M.C. Martin, and M Shivanandan, eds. Washington, DC: International Federation for Family Life Promotion.

———. 1985. "Continuation and effectiveness of contraceptive practice: A cross-sectional approach." *Studies in Family Planning* 16(3):138–153.

———. 1986. "Periodic abstinence in the Philippines: New findings from a national survey." *Regional Research Papers, South and East Asia*. Bangkok, Thailand: The Population Council.

Lubis, F., J. Prihartono, T. Agoestina, B. Affandi, H. Sutedi. 1983. "One-year experience with NORPLANT® implants in Indonesia." *Stud-*

ies in *Family Planning* 14(6/7):181–184.

Marangoni, P., S. Cartagena, J. Alvarado, J. Diaz, and A. Faúndes. 1983. "NORPLANT® implants and the Tcu200 IUD: A comparative study in Ecuador." *Studies in Family Planning* 14(6):177–180.

Mason, K. O. 1970. "A Feasibility Study of the Cost-Effectiveness of Alternative Strategies for Disseminating the Oral Contraceptive in NESA Countries." Research Triangle Park, North Carolina: Research Triangle Institute.

Mauldin, W. P., D. Nortman, and F. F. Stephan. 1967. "Retention of IUDs: An international comparison." *Studies in Family Planning* 1(18):1–12.

Meade, C. W., L. Casarin, M. Diaz, A. Aquado, L. Zacarias, S. Holck, P. Diethelm, J. Annus. 1984. "A clinical study of Norethisterone ethanate in rural Mexico." *Studies in Family Planning* 15(3): 143–148.

Moots, B. L. and H. C. Chen. 1973. "Preliminary report of Taichung IUD4 Study." *Taiwan Population Studies Working Paper* No. 22. Ann Arbor: University of Michigan Population Studies Center.

Moreno, L. 1991. "Differentials in contraceptive failure rates in developing countries: Results from the Demographic and Health Surveys." *Demographic and Health Surveys World Conference*, vol.I:695–716.

Moreno, L. and N. Goldman. 1991. "Contraceptive failure rates in developing countries: Evidence from the Demographic and Health Surveys." *International Family Planning Perspectives* 17(2): 44–49.

Narkavonnakit, T., T. Bennett, and T.R. Balakrishnan. 1982. "Continuation of injectable contraceptives in Thailand." *Studies in Family Planning* 13(4):99–105.

Pariani, S., D. Heer, and M. Van Arsdol. 1987. "Continued contraceptive use in five family planning clinics in Surabaya, Indonesia." *Studies in Family Planning* 22(6):384–390.

Park, I. and S. Kong. 1987. "Contraceptive failure and discontinuation in Korea." In *Comparative Study of Fertility Control Experiences in the Republic of Korea and the Republic of China*. Seoul: Korea Institute for Population and Health.

Phillips, J. 1978. "Continued use of contraceptives among Philippine family planning acceptors." *Studies in Family Planning* 9(7):182–192.

Porter, E. 1984. "Birth control discontinuance as a diffusion process." *Studies in Family Planning* 15(1):20–29.

Potter, R. G., L. P. Chow, C. H. Lee, and A. K. Jain. 1967. "Taiwan: IUD Effectiveness in the Taichung Medical Follow-up Study." *Studies in Family Planning* 1(18):13–24.

Rahman, M., J. Akbar, and J. Phillips. 1990. "Sex composition of children and contraceptive use in Matlab, Bangladesh." Unpublished.

Ross, J.A., A. Germain, J.E. Forrest, and J. Van Ginneken. 1972. "Findings from family planning research." *Reports on Population/Family Planning* 12:1–47.

Ross, J.A., S. Hong, and D. Huber. 1985. *Voluntary Sterilization: An International Factbook*. New York: Association for Voluntary Sterilization.

Ross, J.A., M. Rich, J.P. Molzan. 1989. *Management Strategies for Family Planning Programs*. New York: Columbia University.

Russell-Brown, P., C. Piedrahita, R. Foldesy, M. Steiner, and J. Townsend. 1992. "Comparison of condom breakage during human use with performance in laboratory testing." *Contraception* 45:429–437.

Salah, M., A.G. Ahmed, M. Abo-Eloyoun, and M.M. Shaaban. 1987. "Five year experience with NORPLANT® implants in Assiut, Egypt." *Contraception* 35(6):543–550.

Salem, H.T., M. Salah, M.Y. Aly, A.I. Thabet, M.M. Shaaban, and M.F. Fathalla. 1988. "Acceptability of injectable contraceptives in Assiut, Egypt." *Contraception* 38(6): 697–710.

Shaaban, M., M. Salah, A. Zarzour, and S. Abdullah. 1983. "A prospective study of NORPLANT® implants and the TCu380ag IUD in Assiut, Egypt." *Studies in Family Planning* 14(6/7):163–169.

Sivin, I. 1988. "International experience with NORPLANT® and NORPLANT-2® contraceptives." *Studies in Family Planning* 19(2): 81–94.

———. 1991. "Dose- and age-dependent ectopic pregnancy risks with intrauterine contraception." *Obstetrics and Gynecology* 78(2): 291–298.

———. 1993. Personal communication.

Sivin, I. and F. Schmidt. 1987. "Effectiveness of IUDs: A review." *Contraception* 36(1): 55–84.

Somboonsuk, A., N. Xuto, R.H. Gray, R.A. Grossman. 1978. "A field study of the choice and continuity of use of three contraceptive methods in a rural area of Thailand." *Journal of Biosocial Science* 10(2):209–216.

Teachman, J., H. Suyono, J. Parsons, and I. Rohadi. 1980. "Continuation of contraception on Java-Bali: Preliminary results from the Quarterly Acceptor Survey." *Studies in Family Planning* 11(4):134–144.

Tietze, C. 1967. "Intra-uterine contraception: Research report." *Studies in Family Planning* 1(18):20–24.

Trussell, J. and K. Kost. 1987. "Contraceptive failure in the United States: A critical review of the literature." *Studies in Family Planning* 18(5):237–283.

Westoff, C. 1988. "Contraceptive paths toward the reduction of unintended pregnancy and abortion." *Family Planning Perspectives* 20(1):4–13.

World Health Organization. 1990. "The TCu380A, TCu220C, Multiload 250 and Nova T IUDs at 3, 5 and 7 years of use: Results from three randomized multicentre trials." *Contraception* 42(2):141–158.

Zetina-Lozano, G. 1983. "Menstrual bleeding expectations and short-term contraceptive discontinuation in Mexico." *Studies in Family Planning* 14(5):127–133.

Chapter 8

STERILIZATION

Sterilization[1] offers both advantages and disadvantages compared with other contraceptive methods.

Advantages

Among all contraceptive methods, sterilization offers the longest continuation rate and the lowest failure rate. It is a one-step method with few side effects. For females, the modern techniques of laparoscopic and minilap sterilization permit outpatient procedures under local anesthesia; these have reduced costs, operator time, and medical trauma, and have greatly expanded the use of sterilization internationally.

Disadvantages

Because of its permanency, sterilization is appropriate only for persons who are certain that they want no more children. Some of those adopting it later regret doing so, due to new marriages, the death of a child, or other causes. It is a surgical technique, with the attendant risks which, however, are much lower than the medical risks of repeated pregnancies, induced abortions, and deliveries in most developing countries.

PREVALENCE

1. **Internationally, the prevalence of sterilization is higher than that of any other contraceptive method, but countries and regions vary greatly in its use.**

   1.a. In the developing world over one-fifth (22 percent) of all married women of reproductive age (MWRA) rely on sterilization, (*Tables 1 and 2*). This represents nearly one-half (44 percent) of all contraceptive users. In developed countries 11 percent of MWRA use sterilization, which represents 18 percent of all contraceptive users. Globally, the figures are 20 percent of MWRA and 38 percent of all users, respectively (1990 estimates).

   In the developing world the IUD comes next after sterilization, with 12 percent of MWRA using it (due heavily to its high prevalence in China.) Next is the pill, at 6 percent of MWRA.

   1.b. Regions vary widely in sterilization use, from 37 percent of MWRA in East Asia to over 20 percent in South Asia and Latin America, to fewer than 3 percent in the Middle East/North Africa and sub-Saharan Africa (*Table 1*).

   1.c. In terms of numbers, as of 1990, 169 million MWRA in the developing world used sterilization, and 22 million did so in developed countries, for a total of 191 million women (or spouses).

   1.d. Sterilization users, in absolute numbers, are remarkably concentrated geographically. China has nearly half of all users of sterilization in the developing world and India has over a fourth, while the next country, Brazil, has only 5 percent (*Table 2*). Many African and Middle Eastern countries have only negligible numbers.

   1.e. In percentage terms, 45–50 percent of MWRA use sterilization in South Korea and Puerto Rico; over one-third do so in China and in some Central American countries, and about 30 percent do so in India, Brazil, Thailand, and Sri Lanka. Sterilization is little used in the Middle East and Africa, except for Tunisia (11 percent of MWRA), Kenya (5 percent overall and 8 percent in some population subgroups), and Botswana (5 percent).

   1.f. Globally, vasectomy plays a minor role compared with female sterilization; in *Table 1* female users exceed male users by over three to one worldwide. In essentially every country (except perhaps the Netherlands), female sterilization prevalence exceeds that of vasectomy, especially outside Asia. Vasectomy is important in China (10 percent of couples in 1985), India (11 percent in 1982), and South Korea (11 percent in 1988). For developed countries it is an important method in the United States, Canada, and the United Kingdom (12–14 percent in 1988, 1984, and 1989, respectively); the Netherlands (11 percent in 1988) (Liskin et al., 1992); and New Zealand (23 percent in a 1983–86 study). The dominance of female sterilization may reflect women's greater motivation to contracept, the failure of providers to make vasectomy widely and easily available, and certain cultural constraints; all of these vary by country and region. In Latin America reasons given for the near absence of male sterilization go beyond presumed cultural attitudes; commentators there often cite the failure of providers to offer the method even

Table 1 Percentage of married women of reproductive age using contraception, by method, according to region, 1990 estimates

Method	World	MDCs[b]	LDCs[a]	East Asia	South Asia	Middle East/ North Africa	Sub-Saharan Africa	Latin America
Sterilization	20.1	11.4	22.3	36.5	20.8	1.9	1.2	21.6
Female	15.7	7.6	17.8	28.5	16.0	1.8	1.2	21.0
Male	4.4	3.8	4.5	8.0	4.8	0.1	0.0	0.6
IUD	10.9	5.4	12.3	29.4	4.6	8.1	1.0	6.6
Hormonal	8.6	14.4	7.1	3.9	6.7	12.2	4.4	18.4
Pill	7.7	14.3	6.0	3.7	5.0	12.0	3.0	17.2
Injectables	0.9	0.1	1.1	0.2	1.7	0.2	1.4	1.2
Condom	5.4	15.1	2.9	2.6	3.9	2.9	0.4	2.6
Other	8.0	16.1	5.9	2.2	7.1	11.3	5.1	11.1
Total	53.0	62.4	50.5	74.6	43.1	36.4	12.1	60.3

[a] LDCs = less developed countries, as defined by the United Nations.
[b] MDCs = more developed countries, as defined by the United Nations.
Source: Population Council Data Bank; based upon most recent survey data.

though it is far less costly and invasive than female procedures. Where providers have offered the method and encouraged its use, adoption rates have increased. (See Chapter 6 for the relation of sterilization adoption rates to payments; males may respond more sensitively to payments than do females, who often obtain sterilization in the period soon after a birth.)

STERILIZATION DYNAMICS

2. **Annual adoption rates of sterilization are low, and are considerably lower than for most alternative contraceptive methods, yet sterilization prevalence can rise to a high level.**

   2.a. Annual adoption rates vary from 0–3 percent of all MWRA. In the 17 largest developing countries, with 81 percent of the developing world's population, the annual adoption rate averages 2.3 percent of MWRA per year (average weighted by population size). In 14 smaller countries, the rate is about 2 percent. The remaining developing countries, most of them small, have negligible rates.

3. **Despite low annual adoption rates, the prevalence of sterilization use has risen to over one-fifth of all couples.**

   3.a. This seeming contradiction, of low adoption rates but high prevalence, is explained by four factors that characterize sterilization:

   * Its long continuation rate, of about 15 years, running from about age 30 (the average time of adoption) to about age 45 (an average time for leaving the reproductive age group).

   * Its negligible failure rate, so that few users drop out due to accidental pregnancy.

   * Its long history of availability in many countries, permitting a gradual buildup of users over the years.

   * Its wide age spread at adoption, with many relatively young adopters, so that most of those starting on the method remain in the pool of users many years and contribute to the buildup of users.

Table 2 Number and percentage of married women of reproductive age using sterilization, percentage using any contraceptive method, and percentage of all users who rely on sterilization, by selected countries, 1990 estimates

	Country	No. of MWRA sterilized (000s)	Percent sterilized	Percent using any method	Percent of all users sterilized
1	China	82,582	36.9	74.9	49.2
2	India	51,861	30.9	44.9	68.8
3	Brazil	7,909	29.7	69.2	42.9
4	South Korea	3,639	47.6	76.1	62.5
5	Mexico	3,146	21.4	57.9	37.0
6	Thailand	2,796	30.4	73.5	41.3
7	Bangladesh	2,428	11.0	32.9	33.4
8	Indonesia	1,188	3.6	52.2	6.9
9	Philippines	1,135	12.2	48.9	25.0
10	Colombia	1,037	18.8	66.7	28.2
11	North Korea	992	22.3	68.4	32.7
12	Taiwan	950	26.0	78.0	33.3
13	Argentina	917	19.9	61.5	32.4
14	Pakistan	837	4.2	15.4	27.3
15	Sri Lanka	830	31.4	65.5	47.9
16	Myanmar	752	12.0	45.5	26.4
17	Nepal	585	15.5	18.1	85.5
18	Iran	574	6.3	30.8	20.6
19	South Africa	511	9.4	56.3	16.7
20	Dominican Republic	407	36.5	55.3	66.1
	All developing countries	169,000	22.3	50.5	44.2

Source: Ross, 1992.

PERSONAL CHARACTERISTICS OF USERS

The personal characteristics of sterilization users are fairly consistent for family size, age, sex, and residence, but vary by socioeconomic status.

Number of Living Children, Age, and Sex

4. Sterilization use is most prevalent in families of intermediate sizes.

    4.a. Internationally, sterilization is very little used by those with no or one child. However, in many countries its use is appreciable among those with two children, and it rises thereafter quite sharply among those with three and even four children. At five or more children, adoption of sterilization usually falls off, reflecting partly the circularity that the very absence of sterilization helps to produce larger families.

5. Sterilization use is most prevalent at intermediate ages, following a pattern that is rather consistent across countries, even though countries differ considerably in age at marriage and age at first birth.

    5.a. Age patterns of users are rather consistent across countries, partly for counterbalancing reasons. In countries like India and Bangladesh, women marry and have children quite early but adopt sterilization later in marriage, whereas in societies like China and South Korea, women marry later but adopt sterilization soon afterwards. Generally, sterilization prevalence is substantial at ages 25–29 and rises through ages 35–39, tending to fall off thereafter, since older women experienced much childbearing before simple sterilization techniques became available and during more conservative times.

    Ages for *adopters* of sterilization are below those for *current users*; adopters generally average about age 30, but are younger where sterilization prevalence is high and older where it is low (see Rutenberg and Landry, 1991, *Figure 2*).

6. Nearly everywhere, female sterilization is more prevalent than male sterilization (see section 1.f.).

Residence, Socioeconomic Status, Psychological, and Social-Psychological Variables

7. Rural couples use sterilization about as much as do urban ones.

    7.a. Rural prevalence equals or exceeds urban prevalence in 10 of 23 national surveys (principally DHS surveys; summarized in Ross, 1991, Table 4). This may reflect general modernization or rural program efforts, or both, as in Bangladesh, South Korea, Sri Lanka, Tunisia, Botswana, and Colombia.

8. Sterilization use by socioeconomic status follows no consistent pattern, at least not according to educational attainment.

    8.a. Philliber and Philliber (1985), who reviewed 56 studies from the 1970s and early 1980s, found some consistency of pattern within geographic regions, but that has since disappeared. In 23 recent national surveys socioeconomic patterns are mixed and inconsistent within each region; in some cases sterilization prevalence rises with education level, in others it falls, and in some it follows a partial U-shaped pattern.

9. Studies examining psychological and social-psychological correlates of sterilization have been found to be weak on methodology and to show inconclusive results (see Philliber and Philliber, 1985, Table 1). A review of factors affecting the choice of sterilization (Bulatao, 1989) notes widely varying influences. The economic costs of children are commonly cited, but a variety of psychological elements also come into play in different settings.

DEMOGRAPHIC EFFECTS

10. Sterilization averts large numbers of induced abortions and unwanted births.

    10.a. Most MWRA adopting sterilization have two to four children and are age 30, on average. Without reliable protection from pregnancy over the ensuing years, they would experience substantial numbers of additional pregnancies, induced abortions, and unwanted births. (Estimates for births averted by sterilization are reviewed in Ross et al., 1985.)

    10.b. In South Korea, sterilization use was estimated to avert 540 abortions and 300 births (840 pregnancies) per 1,000 women by the 25th year of marriage (Westoff et al., 1980).

    10.c. The average family size of sterilization adopters has steadily declined over the years; consequently, sterilization has increased its contribution to averting conceptions, induced abortions, and births (Ross et al., 1985, Table E; and Ross et al., 1988, Table 25).

    10.d. Younger cohorts of couples are adopting sterilization earlier than older cohorts did. This pattern holds in nearly all 18 countries with non-negligible sterilization rates. Cohort differences are sharper and appear at earlier ages in countries where overall rates are higher. *Figure 1* shows cohort trends for six high-sterilization countries (Rutenberg and Landry, 1991, analyzing DHS national surveys).

11. **Of those adopting sterilization, the proportion who regret having done so is low overall but higher in certain subgroups.**

11.a. For female sterilization, one review of the literature identifies these subgroups as being women who are young; not married or married fewer than five years; who have only one or two children; who lack a child of each sex; who feel little control over the sterilization decision; and who have husbands opposed to the decision (or who subsequently change partners or experience a child death). However, these are also the subgroups with the lowest adoption rates; in national surveys the overall regret rate is low. Careful counseling reduces the likelihood of regret and points to alternative methods of contraception for sterilization candidates who are unsure (Church and Geller, 1990).

12. **Future sterilization patterns will parallel those prevailing now.**

12.a. Most future sterilization adopters and users will be located where they have been in the past. China and India together have over three-fourths of all sterilization users; because of their size and the well-established role of sterilization there, those countries will continue to dominate the global picture. Other, smaller countries with high sterilization prevalence will continue to have high prevalence, due to the carryover effect of current users and to the established role of the method within their populations.

12.b. Projections for sterilization are more reliable than for other methods, for four reasons: (1) the large body of current users is a known quantity, since national surveys cover over 85 percent of the population of the developing world and over 90 percent of contraceptive users; (2) the relatively young age distribution of adopters and users means they will persist into the future; (3) differential adoption rates by country are fairly stable; and (4) 15-year projections are reliable for the numbers of women of reproductive age, since all are already born.

12.c. These four factors, used in cohort projections and for individual countries, yield an estimate of approximately 158 million sterilizations in the developing world during the 1990–2000 decade, of which China will account for half (*Table 3*).

LEGAL ASPECTS

13. **Sterilization is legal on request in many countries; in others it is legal with restrictions.**

13.a. In one listing of 55 countries, only five make sterilization entirely illegal with no exceptions; seven

Table 3 Sterilization projections for six regions

Projection, year	East Asia	South Asia	Middle East/ North Africa	Sub-Saharan Africa	Central America	South America	Total
Acceptance rate (%)							
1990–95	2.37	2.64	0.20	0.20	1.90	2.18	1.94[a]
1995–2000	2.32	2.46	0.20	0.20	1.86	2.12	1.88[a]
No. of acceptors (000s)							
1990–95	37,233	30,160	440	725	2,238	4,923	75,719
1995–2000	41,858	31,906	514	846	2,567	5,420	83,111
Total	79,091	62,066	954	1,571	4,805	10,343	158,830
No. of users (000s)							
1990	94,803	57,859	790	1,111	4,527	12,238	171,328
1995	120,207	81,269	1,037	1,599	6,241	15,675	226,028
2000	139,347	100,027	1,242	2,100	7,688	18,105	268,509
Increase (no.)	44,544	42,168	452	989	3,161	5,867	97,181
Increase (%)	47.0	72.9	57.2	89.0	69.8	47.9	56.7
No. of MWRA (000s)							
1990	314,014	228,359	43,626	73,462	23,543	45,166	728,170
1995	360,234	259,116	51,139	85,762	27,542	51,061	834,854
2000	392,189	291,100	59,348	100,775	31,560	56,811	931,783
Increase (no.)	78,175	62,741	15,722	27,313	8,017	11,645	203,613
Increase (%)	24.9	27.5	36.0	37.2	34.1	25.8	28.0

[a] Five year acceptors divided by average no. of MWRA, divided by 5.
Note: At the outset the 1990–95 schedule of age-specific acceptance rates is set at a level that, together with the age distribution of nonsterilized married women, will reproduce the overall rate. That schedule of age-specific rates is kept constant for the 1995–2000 period.
Source: Ross, 1992.

Figure 1 Percentage sterilized by exact age among various age cohorts in high prevalence countries

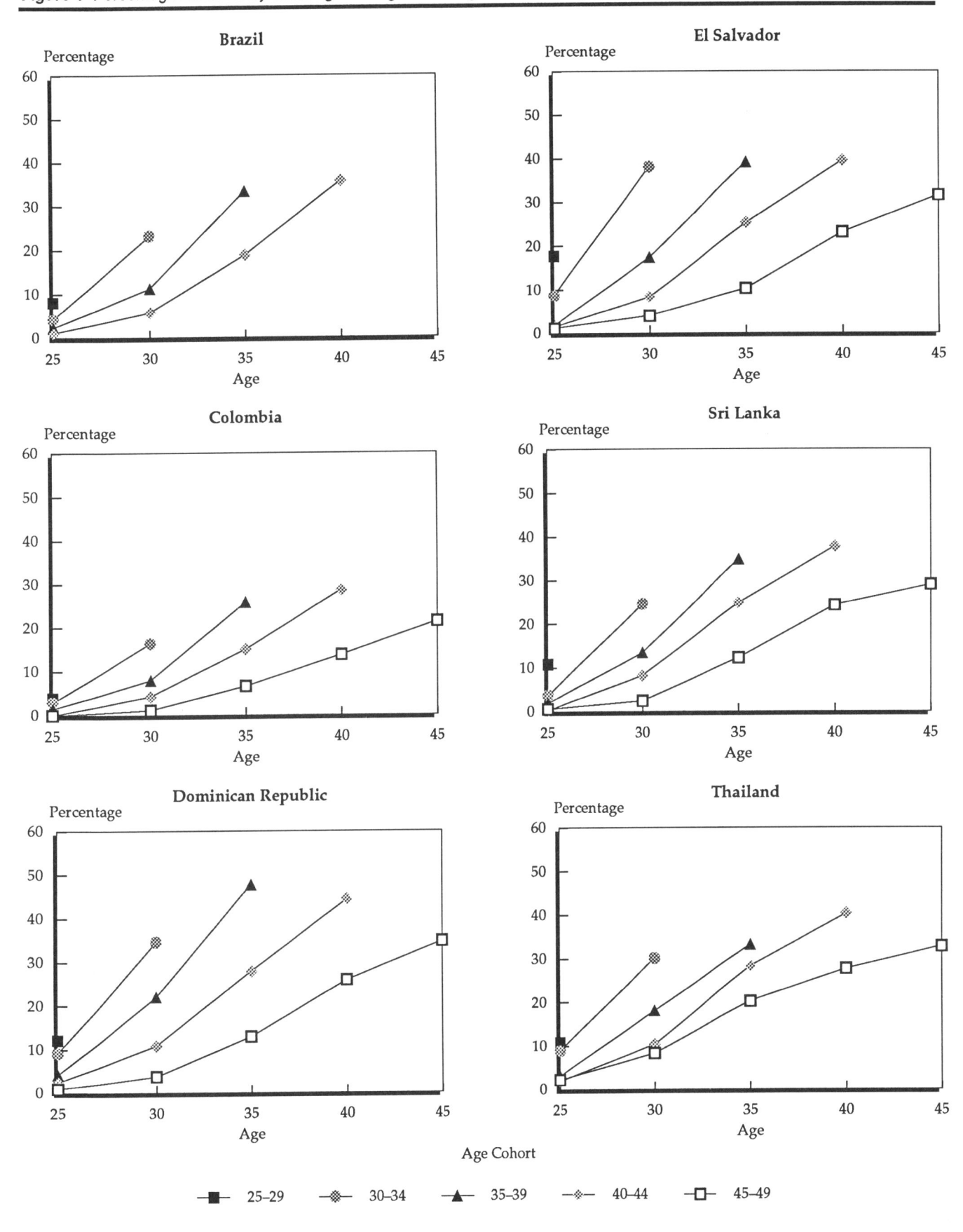

Age Cohort

■ 25–29   ❋ 30–34   ▲ 35–39   ✦ 40–44   ☐ 45–49

Source: Rutenberg and Landry, 1991, Table 1A, p. 689.

more permit it only to save the life of the woman. At the other extreme, 31 countries make it legal simply on request and seven more permit it for eugenic or health reasons. Five countries have no relevant law but do not appear to allow sterilization for contraceptive purposes. (Seven countries with no relevant law still appear to allow it for contraceptive purposes and are included with the 31 that make it legal on request.) Thus, while most of these countries permit sterilization for one reason or another, their laws vary a good deal in restrictiveness. Nevertheless well over half of these countries make sterilization legal on request. In the world as a whole as of 1983, 73 percent of the entire population lived where sterilization was legal with no restrictions or only minor ones, or where in practice it was allowed for contraceptive purposes (see Ross et al., 1992, Table 17; and Ross et al., 1985, Table 3.2).

13.b. The actual availability of sterilization services is more limited than the above numbers imply. Besides the complete absence of services in many areas, nearly all countries set conditions on access to sterilization. Usually a woman must have a minimum number of children, most often two but sometimes three or more. Some countries also set age limits; these range from age 21 or 22 to age 25, 30, and older. Most countries specify that the procedure must be performed by a physician, and many require approval of the spouse for female sterilization.

13.c. Liberalization of laws and conditions governing sterilization occurred during the decades of the 1970s and 1980s (Vumbaco, 1976; Stepan et al., 1981; Isaacs and Cook, 1984).

MORBIDITY AND MORTALITY

See Chapter 12 for evidence on morbidity and mortality associated with male and female sterilization.

NOTES

1. Findings for this section are drawn from Ross (1992) where not otherwise stated. Detailed references to national surveys and other data sources appear there.

REFERENCES

Bulatao, R. A. 1989. "Toward a framework for understanding contraceptive method choice." In *Choosing a Contraceptive: Method Choice in Asia and the United States*. R.A. Bulatao, J.A. Palmore, and S.E. Ward (eds). Boulder: Westview Press. Pp. 277–304.

Church, C.A. and J.S. Geller. 1990. "Voluntary Female Sterilization: Number One and Growing." *Population Reports* Series C, No. 10:1–23.

Isaacs, S.L. and R.J. Cook. 1984. "Laws and Policies Affecting Fertility: A Decade of Change." *Population Reports* 12(6):105–150.

Liskin, L., E. Benoit, and R. Blackburn. 1992. "Vasectomy: New Opportunities." *Population Reports* 20(1), Series D, No. 5:1–23.

Philliber, S.G. and W.W. Philliber. 1985. "Social and psychological perspectives on voluntary sterilization: A review." *Studies in Family Planning* 16(1):1–29.

Ross, J.A. 1992. "Sterilization: Past, present, future." *Studies in Family Planning* 23(3): 187–198.

Ross, J.A., S. Hong, and D.H. Huber. 1985. *Voluntary Sterilization: An International Fact Book*. New York: Association for Voluntary Sterilization.

Ross, J.A., M. Rich, J.P Molzan, and M. Pensak. 1988. *Family Planning and Child Survival: 100 Developing Countries*. New York: Center for Population and Family Health, Columbia University.

Ross, J., W.P. Mauldin, S. Green, and E.R. Cooke. 1992. *Family Planning and Child Survival Programs as Assessed in 1991*. New York: The Population Council.

Rutenberg, N. and E. Landry. 1991. "Use of and demand for sterilization: A comparison of recent findings from the demographic and health surveys." *Demographic and Health Surveys World Conference*. August 5–7. Washington, DC. Vol. 1:667–693.

Stepan, J., E.H. Kellogg, and P.T. Piotrow. 1981. "Legal Trends and Issues in Voluntary Sterilization." *Population Reports* 9(2): Series E, No. 6:73–102.

Vumbaco, B.J. 1976. "Recent law and policy changes in fertility control." *Population Reports* Series E, No. 4:41–51.

Westoff, C.F., N. Goldman, S.E. Khoo, and M.K. Choe. 1980. "The recent demographic history of sterilization in Korea." *International Family Planning Perspectives* 6(4):136–145.

Chapter 9

INDUCED ABORTION

Induced abortion is widely resorted to, whether under legal or illegal conditions. Where it is safe and legal it prevents some unwanted births, depresses fertility rates, and reduces the maternal mortality rate. Where it is illegal and unsafe, however, it increases maternal morbidity and mortality. Abortion has complex interrelations with contraceptive use: The two are often used by the same population subgroups, but contraceptive use at high levels tends to drive out abortions. In the absence of contraceptive alternatives, septic abortions may become so numerous as to account for a substantial proportion of all maternal deaths and constitute a heavy burden on the obstetric capacity of the country.

INCIDENCE OF ABORTION

1. **Globally, abortions occur in substantial numbers, whether legal or not.**

    1.a. In 1987 an estimated 35 to 53 million induced abortions were performed worldwide,[1] amounting to about one-fifth to one-third of births. Between one-fifth and two-fifths of abortions were clandestine (Henshaw, 1990).

2. **Use of induced abortion is common in at least three large regions of the developing world, less so in sub-Saharan Africa and West Asia.**

    2.a. For four regions, *Table 1* shows recent estimates for abortion measures, under alternative assumptions (Frejka, 1993). The table gives only one estimate for East Asia, due to better data there. West Asia is omitted from the table. The table provides demographic effects, which are discussed in section 6 below. (For the methodology used, see Frejka and Atkin, 1990.)

    Numbers of abortions: The sum of the low estimates in column 5, compared to the sum of the high estimates in the column, gives a range of 21.7 to 34.0 million induced abortions per year (midpoint 27.8 million). (The total for developed countries is additional to this.)

    Total abortion rate[2]: A young woman passing through the current rates of abortion for the different ages would have 1.3 abortions in her lifetime in East Asia (column 6), and 1.4 to 2.0 abortions in Latin America. The estimates for South and Southeast Asia, as well as for Africa, are considerably lower.

    Abortion ratio (abortions per 100 live births): Because this ratio reflects the number of births, it responds to contraceptive use as well as to abortion; therefore, the relative positions of the regions may differ from those for the total abortion rate. In terms of the abortion ratio, East Asia ranks higher than Latin America, due perhaps to its very high level of contraceptive use. Again, South and Southeast Asia, and particularly Africa, show considerably less abortion activity than do the other regions. The East Asia rates are elevated partly because of the much more liberal abortion regulations and practices there.

    2.b. In China in the mid-1980s the ratio of abortions to live births was 45–50 per 100 (Wu et al., 1992), a ratio that agrees closely with that for East Asia.

    2.c. The average woman in Brazil and Mexico could expect to undergo 1.5 abortions in her lifetime, vs. 1.3 in Peru in the 1970s (Frejka, 1984), and 2.6 in Cuba in the 1980s (Hollerbach and Diaz-Briquet, 1983).

    2.d. Statistics from Bulgaria, Czechoslovakia, and Yugoslavia (reporting in all three is believed to be nearly complete) indicate that between 40 percent and 50 percent of pregnancies in the mid-1980s ended in abortion. In Romania (1983) and the USSR (1987) (where statistics are incomplete), over 50 percent of pregnancies ended in abortion (Henshaw, 1990).

    2.e. In Japan official statistics indicate that 27 percent of pregnancies ended in abortion in 1987. These numbers are thought to be incomplete. Projections from provinces believed to have complete statistics indicate that over half of all pregnancies ended in abortion in 1975 (Henshaw, 1990).

3. **Data from hospitals in the developing world indicate that increasing numbers of women are seeking either induced abortions or treatment for complications from abortion.**

    3.a. For sub-Saharan Africa, one review of the literature found increasing hospital admissions for abor-

Table 1 Estimates of births averted by contraception and induced abortion, late 1980s

Region	Alternative[a]	Births averted (in millions) Total (1)	Contraception (2)	Induced abortion (3)	Proportion of births averted by induced abortion (in %) (4)	Absolute number of induced abortions (in millions) (5)	Total abortion rate (6)	Abortions per 100 live births (7)
Africa	A	3.3	3.2	0.1	3	0.2	0.05	0.7
	B	4.7	3.2	1.5	32	3.4	0.7	13
East Asia	One only	31.9	24.9	7.0	22	11.9	1.3	53
South and South East Asia	A	23.3	20.7	2.6	11	5.2	0.4	9
	B	26.9	20.7	6.2	23	12.5	0.9	22
Latin America	A	11.2	8.8	2.4	21	4.4	1.4	35
	B	12.2	8.8	3.4	28	6.2	2.0	50

[a] Alternatives A and B were selected to correspond, respectively, to low and high estimates of induced abortion incidence.
Source: Frejka, 1993, Table 1.

tion complications throughout the region in the late 1970s and early 1980s and high rates of maternal deaths due to abortion. Kenyatta National Hospital in Nairobi and Mama Yemo in Kinshasa, which were reporting 2,000 to 3,000 admissions a year for abortion complications in that period, were treating 30 to 60 cases a day by the late 1980s. For Kenyatta Hospital, this was a five-fold increase. The few community-based studies available suggested that the numbers being seen in the hospitals were ". . . only the tip of the iceberg" (Coeytaux, 1988).

3.b. The Khartoum Teaching Hospital in Sudan treated 700 incomplete abortions in 1974, of which at least two-thirds were estimated to have been induced; by 1988 the number had risen to 3,000 incomplete abortion admissions a year. These cases represented 80 percent of emergency ob/gyn admissions (Toubia, 1989).

3.c. In 18 hospitals in Jakarta, Indonesia, the ratio of abortions to live births increased steadily, from 183 per 1,000 in 1972 to 396 per 1,000 in 1975 (Samil, 1989). The ratio of abortions to births rose dramatically in Ramathibodi Hospital in Bangkok. In 1975 the abortion ratio was less than 10 abortions per 1,000 live births; by 1979 the ratio was 258 abortions per 1,000 live births (Chaturachinda et al., 1981).

CHARACTERISTICS OF ABORTION CLIENTS[3]

Marital Status

4. In Asia married women seek abortions more frequently than do unmarried women. In parts of Africa, abortion clients are more likely to be unmarried.

4.a. In Jakarta, Indonesia, 97 percent of women seeking abortions in hospitals were married. Married women account for the majority of abortions reported in studies from other parts of the country as well (Samil, 1989). The majority of abortion clients in India and Bangladesh are married (Liskin, 1980; Royston and Armstrong, 1989). In a Philippine study, 75 percent of women who underwent abortions were married, 20 percent were single, and the remainder were widowed, divorced, or separated (Gallen, 1982).

4.b. In Nigeria women seeking abortions are often unmarried (Ovin et al., 1984; Mashabala, 1989). A study of hospital records from Benin City revealed that 71 percent of induced abortions were among primary and secondary school students, of whom only 9.8 percent were married (Nnatu, 1988).

4.c. In Shanghai rates of abortion during the 1980s increased faster for teenagers than for older women, although rates still remained higher for older women than for teenagers. In 1988 three-quarters of abortion recipients were married. Single women tended to seek abortions later in pregnancy than did married women (Wu et al., 1992).

Age and Parity

5. Where married women constitute the main group undergoing abortion, clients are older and have two or more children. Where unmarried women predominate, clients are younger and more often have no children. However, these patterns are quite variable across countries and regions.

5.a. In Indonesia (Jakarta), India, and the Philippines, the average age of abortion patients ranged from 28 to 31 (Samil, 1989; Gallen, 1982). Average ages for clients, across abortion practitioners in a Thailand study, ranged from 18 to 43 (Narkavonnakit, 1979).

5.b. Half of the Indonesian abortion patients were pregnant for at least the fifth time (Samil, 1989). The average parity of Bangladeshi women was four; Filipino women had an average of 2.9 living children (Khan et al., 1984; Gallen, 1982). Averages for the number of living children among clients of various practitioners in Thailand ranged from 2.2 to 7.4 (Narkavonnakit, 1979).

5.c. In Jamalpur, Bangladesh, abortion ratios were three times higher among women over 35 and women with five or more children than among women below age 25 or those who were childless (Khan et al., 1984).

5.d. One-quarter of women admitted to Botswana hospitals for treatment related to abortion in 1976 were under 18 years old. In Sierra Leone (1980) 23 percent of abortions were to teenagers (Mashabala, 1989).

DEMOGRAPHICS OF ABORTION

6. Liberalization of abortion laws and increased use of induced abortion can help produce a decline in a country's birth rate, but abortion is only one factor limiting fertility.

    6.a. *Demographic effects*: Columns 1–4 of *Table 1* provide estimates of total births averted (in millions) due to the use of contraception and induced abortion, as well as the proportion of births averted due to abortion. That proportion is one-fifth to one-fourth in East Asia and Latin America, lower in South and Southeast Asia, and rather indeterminate in Africa, where data are especially poor. It is estimated that abortion averted about seven million births annually in the late 1980s in East Asia, fewer in South and Southeast Asia, considerably fewer in Latin America (due to its much smaller population), and even fewer in Africa.

    6.b. In most industrialized countries declines in fertility steepened after liberalization of abortion laws. In Hungary, for example, the pace of the fertility decline increased substantially after legalization of abortion in 1955 (Tietze, 1964). In general, fertility decline began long before laws changed and almost certainly would have continued without the change in abortion laws (Tietze and Henshaw, 1986), although probably not as rapidly.

    6.c. A pattern of declining birth rates after legalization of abortion was observed in many East European countries. Nearly all these countries legalized abortion about 1955, after which their birth rates fell substantially more than did those in Western European countries. The decline also exceeded those in East Germany and Albania, where abortion remained illegal for some years (Tietze, 1964).

    6.d. When several Eastern European countries restricted access to abortion by repealing long-standing liberal abortion laws, fertility increased. Romania reversed its liberal abortion policy in 1966: The birth rate rose from 12.8 per 1,000 population in December 1966 to 39.9 per 1,000 in September 1967, and began to decline gradually thereafter (see *Figure 1*).

    6.e. Abortion is credited for a portion of Japan's fertility decline (Davis, 1963).

7. In the early stages of the fertility transition, abortion rates (per woman, not necessarily per pregnancy) tend to rise. Later, as effective use of modern methods of contraception increases, abortion rates may fall. (Note: Survey counts of numbers of abortions are nearly always too low and must be interpreted cautiously.)

    7.a. The proportion of Taiwanese women who had ever used contraception rose from 28 percent to 76 percent between 1965 and 1976. Over the same period the proportion of women who admitted having undergone an abortion rose from 9 percent to 21 percent (Royston and Armstrong, 1989).

    7.b. In the 1950s Japan experienced a dramatic drop in the number of births per 1,000 women of reproductive age. The rate declined by 41 percent between 1950 and 1957, in large part because of abortion (Davis, 1963). The reported number of abortions in Japan rose from 246,000 in 1949 to 1.2 million in 1955, then dropped to 568,000 by 1983. Over the same period the total fertility rate declined from around 4.5 to 1.8 children per woman (Anon., 1987).

    7.c. In South Korea the birth rate fell by 30 percent between 1960 and 1968, while the proportion of pregnancies reported to have ended in abortion rose from 6 percent to 21 percent (Royston and Armstrong, 1989). Between 1973 and 1979 both the abortion rate and the contraceptive prevalence rate increased rapidly. After 1979, contraceptive prevalence continued to rise but the abortion rate fell back to its 1983 level (Henshaw, 1990).

    7.d. In China the level of abortion is now substantially lower than it was in 1983. France, Italy, and Japan have all reported recent declines in use of abortion, probably as a result of increased use of modern contraceptives (Henshaw, 1990).

Figure 1 Crude birth rate, abortion mortality rate, and maternal mortality rate in relation to the Romanian anti-abortion law of 1966

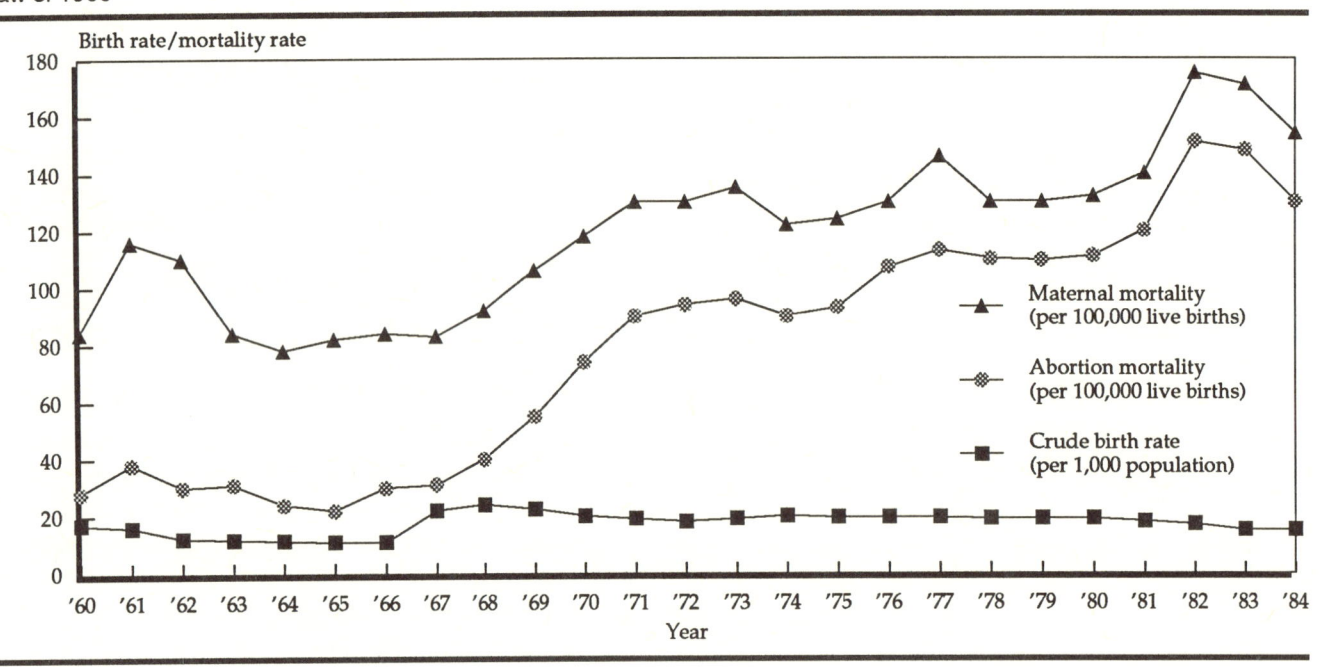

Source: Royston and Armstrong, 1989, Figure 6.2.

8. **Contraceptive use cannot completely eliminate induced abortion in its role as a backup means of avoiding unwanted births, since no contraceptive is 100 percent effective.**

   8.a. Even if 90 percent of couples aim for a two-child family 1by using 90 percent effective contraception, the average woman can expect 1.7 abortions within the course of her life (Tietze and Bongaarts, 1975).

   8.b. Probably no population has lowered its total fertility rate to 2.2 or less without recourse to induced abortion. Population stabilization without use of induced abortion is improbable unless major changes in contraceptive technology or sexual behavior occur (Tietze and Bongaarts, 1975).

9. **One hundred abortions prevent fewer than one hundred births.**

   9.a. Even when the number of induced abortions equals the number of live births (as in Hungary in 1959), the birth rate will not necessarily be halved, since 100 aborted pregnancies account for less exposure time than do 100 full-term pregnancies (Potter, 1963; World Health Organization, 1970). That is, abortions can occur much more often than births can.

   9.b. The combination of induced abortion and effective contraception comes much closer to averting one birth than does abortion alone. Furthermore, fewer abortions are necessary to produce a given birth rate, since fewer pregnancies occur. In a noncontracepting population 100 induced abortions avert only 30–45 live births, depending on the length of lactation. In a population that contracepts with 90 percent effectiveness, 100 abortions avert 72–82 births (Potter, 1963).

Contraceptive Use

10. **Women highly motivated to control their fertility tend to use both contraception and abortion.**

    10.a. The positive relationship between use of abortion and contraceptive use has been documented in Brazil, Israel, Taiwan, the Philippines, Singapore, and Turkey (Liskin, 1980).

    10.b. Only 12 percent of noncontraceptors in South Korea had experienced an abortion, compared with 46 percent of contraceptors (1971 data). Of women who had ever obtained an abortion, 73 percent were using contraception, while only 29 percent of women who had never had an abortion were currently contracepting (Tietze and Henshaw, 1986).

    10.c. Of 115 Filipino women who reported having had abortions, 70 percent had ever used contraception. Only 33 percent of the 561 respondents who had never had an abortion had used contraception. Of 269 contracepting women, 30 percent had also experienced an abortion, but only 8 percent of 407 noncontracepting women had used abortion (Flavier and Chen, 1980).

11. **Contraceptive use often increases following an abortion; however, postabortion services are inadequate.**

   11.a. Barriers to postabortion counselling and contraceptive services include legal problems, separation of abortion and family planning facilities, and an absence of motivation among some doctors to help women avoid unwanted pregnancies. Expert recommendations are that a range of contraceptive methods be made available at all abortion facilities, and that clinically all methods are appropriate assuming no medical contraindications and careful counselling (Technical Working Group, 1993).

   11.b. Only 25 percent of Indian women hospitalized for complications of induced abortion used contraceptives prior to the abortion, but 88 percent adopted a method afterwards. Of 301 Thai women undergoing an abortion, only 4 percent had used contraception before the procedure, but 44 percent adopted a method afterwards (Royston and Armstrong, 1989).

   11.c. Among Filipino women who had an abortion, only 31 percent had been using contraception immediately prior to becoming pregnant, whereas 61 percent were using modern methods at the time of the interview (Gallen, 1982).

   11.d. Several studies in India comment on the frequency with which women undergoing abortion adopt either an IUD or sterilization (Chhabra et al., 1988; Khan et al., 1990); abortions and sterilizations are often performed in the same operating session. According to official estimates, 29 percent of abortions are accompanied by sterilization (Henshaw, 1990).

   11.e. In Cubuk, Turkey, women who had undergone an abortion were three times more likely to switch to a more effective method of contraception than were women who had not undergone an abortion (Bulut, 1984).

LEGALITY OF ABORTION

12. **The extent to which abortion is legal differs greatly from country to country (see *Table 2*). Common restrictions include parental notification for minors, gestational age, husband's permission, waiting periods, and counseling.**

   12.a. About 40 percent of the world's population have access to abortion on demand, while another 25 percent live in countries that allow it only when the woman's life is in danger. The remainder live under various restrictions that limit the right to an abortion (Jacobson, 1990; Henshaw, 1990).

   12.b. Government health facilities in China, India, Tunisia, Cuba, and Vietnam provide legal abortions alongside other health care (Henshaw, 1990), although actual availability may vary.

   12.c. In Bangladesh, parts of Indonesia, and Malaysia, abortion is illegal but menstrual regulation is available up to 10–12 weeks after a woman's last period (Henshaw, 1990; Samil, 1989).

   12.d. In most of sub-Saharan Africa abortion is highly restricted. It is illegal except to save a woman's life in many countries. Abortion for reasons other than a woman's physical health is legal in only three countries *(Table 2)*.

13. **The legality of abortion is often a poor indication of its availability.**

   13.a. Abortion may be easy to obtain even if it is only partially legal. In Israel, South Korea, and New Zealand, abortion is illegal for reasons other than maternal health, yet abortion rates in these countries are comparable to those of countries with far less restrictive laws. Most countries in Latin America have restrictive abortion laws but many physicians in major cities will perform abortions and some cities have clinics that specialize in abortion (Henshaw, 1990).

   13.b. Laws that allow abortions to be performed only in hospitals, by highly trained professionals, often cause delays until the pregnancy is more difficult to terminate or the woman resorts to use of nonstandard methods. In Zambia first-trimester abortions are legal but must occur in a hospital with the permission of two physicians and one specialist. In the University Teaching Hospital there, nine women are treated for complications of illegal abortions for every legal abortion performed (Castle et al., 1990; Jacobson, 1990).

   13.c. In India qualified physicians perform legal abortions at some government health facilities, but 14 out of every 15 doctors trained to perform abortions live in cities, while 78 percent of India's population live in rural areas (Jacobson, 1990; Tietze and Henshaw, 1986).

14. **In the past five years most legislation concerning abortion has served to increase rather than restrict its availability.**

Table 2 Countries by restrictiveness of abortion law, according to region, January 1, 1990

Law	Africa	Asia and Oceania	Europe	North America	South America
To save a woman's life	Angola Benin Botswana Burkina Faso Central African Republic Chad Gabon Ivory Coast Libya Madagascar Malawi Mali Mauritania Mauritius Mozambique Niger Nigeria Senegal Somalia Sudan Zaire	Afghanistan Bangladesh Indonesia Iran Iraq Laos Lebanon Myanmar Oman Pakistan Philippines Sri Lanka Syria United Arab Emirates Yemen	Belgium Ireland	Dominican Republic El Salvador*,† Guatemala Haiti Honduras Mexico* Nicaragua Panama	Brazil* Chile Colombia Ecuador* Paraguay Venezuela
Other maternal health reasons	Algeria Cameroon* Congo Egypt† Ethiopia Ghana*,† Guinea Kenya Lesotho Liberia*,† Morocco Namibia*,† Rwanda Sierra Leone South Africa*,† Tanzania Uganda Zimbabwe*,†	Hong Kong*,† Israel*,† Jordan* South Korea*,† Kuwait† Malaysia*,† Mongolia Nepal New Zealand*,† Papua New Guinea Saudi Arabia Thailand*	Albania Northern Ireland Portugal*,† Spain*,† Switzerland	Costa Rica Jamaica Trinidad & Tobago	Argentina* Bolivia* Guyana Peru
Social and social-medical reasons	Burundi Zambia†	Australia† India**,†† Japan*,†,§§ North Korea*,† Taiwan*,†	Bulgaria*,†,‡ Finland*,†,‡,‡‡ West Germany*,†,‡‡,*† Great Britain† Hungary*,†,‡,‡‡ Poland*,§§,‡‡		Uruguay*,§
On request	Togo Tunisia‡‡	China Singapore Turkey§§ Vietnam	Austria‡‡,*† Czechoslovakia‡‡ Denmark‡‡ France§§ East Germany‡‡ Greece‡‡ Italy‡‡ Netherlands Norway‡‡ Romania‡‡ Soviet Union‡‡ Sweden*‡ Yugoslavia††	Canada Cuba†† Puerto Rico United States	

*Includes juridical grounds, such as rape and incest.   †Includes abortion for genetic defects.   ‡Approval is automatic for women who meet certain age, marital, and/or parity requirements.   §Not permitted for health reasons, but may be permitted for serious economic difficulty.   **During the first 20 weeks.   ††During the first 10 weeks.   ‡‡During the first three months or 12 weeks.   §§No formal authorization is required, and abortion is permitted in a doctor's office; thus, abortion is defacto available on request.   *†Gestation limit is for interval since implantation.   *‡During the first 18 weeks.
Notes: Table does not include countries with fewer than one million inhabitants or those for which information on the legal status of abortion is unknown (e.g. Bhutan and Cambodia). All abortions are permitted only prior to fetal viability unless otherwise indicated in footnotes.
Source: Henshaw, 1990, p. 77.

14.a. In 1986 Vietnam removed all mention of abortion from the criminal law codes. In the same year Greece and Czechoslovakia made first-trimester abortion available on request. Smaller countries such as Cape Verde, Cyprus, and French Polynesia have recently liberalized their abortion laws. The United States, Poland, and the Philippines have restricted abortion (Henshaw, 1990).

MEDICAL COMPLICATIONS AND MORTALITY ASSOCIATED WITH ABORTION (See also Chapter 11)

15. Abortion, when performed correctly, is now one of the safest of all surgical procedures, particularly when it occurs in the first trimester of pregnancy, when risks are lowest.

15.a. In the United States death rates from causes related to pregnancy and childbearing are 11 times higher than those from abortion (Henshaw, 1990). In 1977 1.4 deaths resulted from every 100,000 abortions, while 16 people died for every 100,000 tonsillectomies (Liskin, 1980). In Sweden mortality from abortions decreased from 250 deaths per 100,000 abortions in the late 1940s to less than one death per 100,000 abortions in the late 1970s.

15.b. In the United States abortion mortality at eight weeks of gestation is only 0.2 per 100,000 procedures (*Figure 2*). The risk of mortality rises by 20 percent with each additional week of gestation up to 15 weeks, and increases even faster between 15 and 20 weeks (Royston and Armstrong, 1989). At 21 weeks of gestation, abortion mortality is 12.7 per 100,000 procedures (Henshaw, 1990).

15.c. A 1968 survey of 1,890 women in Santiago, Chile, revealed that of women who underwent an abortion at three to five months of gestation, 47 percent were hospitalized for complications. Of women who sought an abortion during the first month of pregnancy, only 18 percent required hospitalization (Royston and Armstrong, 1989).

15.d. Most of the gains in reducing mortality from abortions have occurred at the later gestational ages. In the United States, risks of mortality at gestations of 13–15 weeks dropped by 85 percent during the 1970s, while mortality risks at eight weeks of gestation remained more or less constant (Tietze and Henshaw, 1986).

16. Liberalization of abortion laws has increased the numbers of abortions reported, but decreased the numbers of deaths from abortion.

16.a. In the United States after liberalization of abortion laws in 1973, the number of women dying from postabortion complications fell sharply, even though the number of reported abortions increased (Liskin, 1980). Liberalization of abortion laws results in a rise in the number of safe legal abortions; many of these replace illegal abortions. It is usually unclear how many abortions occurred before liberalization, but a change in laws most likely reduces their numbers.

16.b. In Singapore abortion became available on request in 1974. Between 1968 and 1970, 51 out of 11,151 known abortions resulted in death. Between 1974 and 1976, only 26 of 40,880 abortion clients died (Royston and Armstrong, 1989).

Complications

17. Many of the admissions to obstetric and gynecological wards of hospitals in developing countries are for treatment of complications of induced abortion. Treating complications of induced abortion imposes severe costs.

17.a. Complications from abortion accounted for 40 percent of admissions to the acute gynecological ward at Kenyatta National Hospital in Nairobi in the

Figure 2 Number of reported maternal deaths per 100,000 induced abortions, by number of weeks of gestation, United States, 1981–85

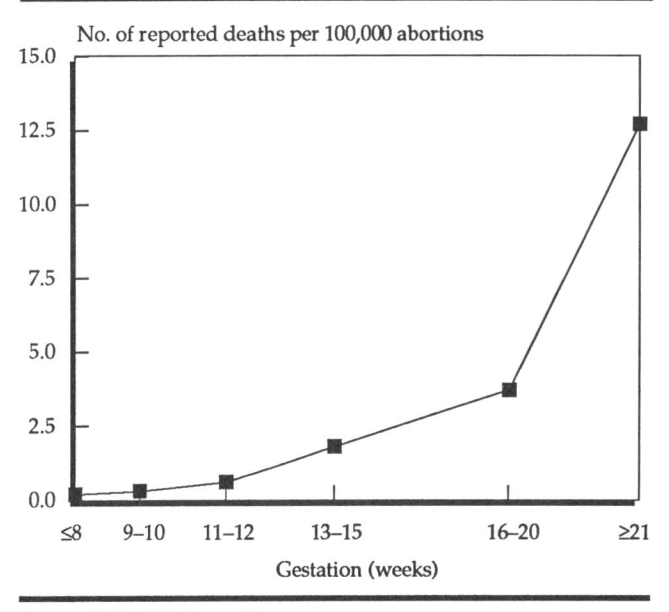

Source: Gold, 1990, Figure 15.
Reproduced with the permission of The Alan Guttmacher Institute from Rachel Benson Gold, *Abortion and Women's Health: A Turning Point for America*, 1990.

early 1980s (Ladipo, 1989). At the University Teaching Hospital in Yaoundé, Cameroon, 32 percent of emergency admissions for obstetric complications were for abortion-related causes (Leke, 1987).

17.b. At the Korle Bu Hospital in Ghana, 60–80 percent of minor operations were performed to correct complications of induced abortion in the early 1970s (Ladipo, 1989).

17.c. Calculations from the Dominican Republic show that treating a complicated abortion case costs 12 times as much as managing a simple delivery (Liskin, 1980). The average illegal abortion treated in Latin American hospitals requires two to three bed days, 15–20 minutes of operating time, antibiotics, anesthesia, and possibly a blood transfusion (Fortney, 1981).

17.d. Hospitals in Latin America and Africa use from 3 percent to 41 percent of their blood supply in treating women with complications from illegal abortions. In Turkey and Venezuela blood transfusions account for nearly half the cost of treatment for abortions (Liskin, 1980; Royston and Armstrong, 1989).

17.e. In the International Postpartum Program of the Population Council, abortion-related cases represented 22 percent of all obstetric-related cases in four Latin American hospitals, 16 percent in three Middle Eastern hospitals, and 10 percent in 11 Far Eastern and South Asian hospitals (Zatuchni, 1970, p.50).

18. **Septic abortion[4] and hemorrhage are the most common complications of abortion, followed by uterine perforation and cervical laceration.**

18.a. In Nairobi in the early 1980s, almost one quarter of the women needing postabortion treatment presented with sepsis (Ladipo, 1989). Of 491 women treated for complications of abortion at the Dhaka Medical College Hospital in Bangladesh, 85 percent of the women who tried to induce an abortion by inserting a solid object into their uterus had developed sepsis. All of the women who tried chemical instillation were infected (Khan et al., 1984).

18.b. Complication rates following first-trimester abortions can be very low. Three clinics in New York City monitored the outcomes of 170,000 first-trimester abortions between 1971 and 1987. Fewer than one patient per 1,000 was hospitalized for suspected perforation, ectopic pregnancy, hemorrhage, sepsis, or incomplete abortion. Fewer than nine patients per 1,000 experienced minor complications (Hakim-Elahi et al., 1990).

18.c. Prolonged or excessive bleeding following an abortion requires a blood transfusion in 2 percent to 45 percent of cases (Ladipo, 1989; Liskin, 1980). Hemorrhages require immediate treatment, which is often difficult because of inadequate blood supplies or facilities for transfusion (Ladipo, 1989).

18.d. Uterine perforation, cervical laceration, chemical burns (from drinking or douching with toxic substances), and internal bleeding (from abdominal massage) are all associated with traditional methods of abortion (Liskin, 1980).

19. **In many developing countries, deaths from septic abortions account for a substantial portion of all maternal deaths.[5]**

19.a. Estimates suggest that abortion-related deaths account for a minimum of 23 percent of all maternal deaths (Royston and Armstrong, 1989). According to one study of 60 developing countries, an estimated 68,000 women died as a result of illegal abortion in 1977 (Rochat et al., 1980).

19.b. In Addis Ababa, Ethiopia, 54 percent of all direct obstetric deaths resulted from complications of criminal abortion (Kwast and Stevens, 1987). Deaths from abortion accounted for a full 86 percent of all maternal deaths in registration data for Romania in 1984 (Royston and Armstrong, 1989).

19.c. In reports for Colombia, Jamaica, and Nigeria, 29 percent, 33 percent, and 35 percent of all maternal deaths, respectively, are from complications of induced abortion (Royston and Armstrong, 1989).

19.d. Septic abortion caused 40 percent of all maternal deaths between 1970 and 1978 in the Maternal and Child Health Institute in Bogota, Colombia (Liskin, 1980).

20. **The legal status and political setting of abortion strongly affects maternal mortality numbers and rates.**

20.a. In the developing world, illegal abortion kills one woman for every 1,000 to 2,000 procedures. In such settings, abortion is 10 to 250 times more dangerous than any method of contraception (Liskin, 1980).

20.b. Both Hungary and Czechoslovakia legalized abortion in the mid 1950s. Between 1953 and 1957, mortality rates from abortion declined 56 percent in Czechoslovakia. Between 1958 and 1962, mortality rates from abortion declined 38 percent in Hungary. No major European or North American country has achieved such a large decline without liberalization of abortion laws (Tietze and Henshaw, 1986).

20.c. After Romania made abortion illegal in 1966, the abortion mortality rate rose to seven times its level when abortion was legal (Tietze and Henshaw, 1986) (see 6.d. and *Figure 1*).

20.d. In the United States the number of deaths from abortion decreased after the abortion law was liberalized in 15 states in 1970 and after the Supreme Court acted in 1973 (Gold, 1990) (see *Figure 3*).

TRADITIONAL METHODS OF ABORTION

Women relied on traditional practitioners and folk methods to terminate unwanted pregnancies long before the development of modern methods. Traditional methods are still common in countries where access to abortion is limited.

21. Inserting objects into the uterus, drinking or douching with special liquids, and abdominal massage are the most common traditional methods of inducing abortion.

21.a. Of the 491 women treated at the Dhaka Medical College Hospital for treatment of complications from induced abortion (see 18.a.), 42 percent had tried an oral abortifacient; 33 percent had inserted objects into the uterus; 8 percent had instilled chemicals into the vagina; and 18 percent had had a modern procedure done elsewhere (Khan et al., 1984).

21.b. In Thailand massage and uterine injection account for over three quarters of traditional abortions. Massage involves locating the fetal mass and pressing the abdomen until bleeding begins. Uterine injection entails dripping a liquid (saline solution, alcohol, gasoline, or a water-cumin mixture) through a catheter into the uterus (Narkavonnakit, 1979).

21.c. In the Philippines abdominal massage and catheter insertion (placing a rubber catheter in the cervix and taping it to the leg in an effort to stimulate bleeding) are traditional methods of abortion. Clients cited catheter insertion as the most common (accounting for almost one-half of procedures), while practitioners reported performing massage more frequently (49 percent of procedures) (Gallen, 1982). Catheter insertion is apparently also common in Latin America and the Caribbean (Frejka et al., 1989).

21.d. Plants are common sources of abortifacients. In the Philippines and Latin America patients boil plant material and drink the resulting liquid (Frejka et al., 1989; Gallen, 1982). Twigs, roots, or bundles of leaves are inserted into the uterus to induce bleeding in Bangladesh and parts of Africa (Islam, 1982; Liskin, 1980). About 20 percent of plants used for these purposes do have abortifacients in them and may be partially effective, according to a WHO study (Frejka et al., 1989).

22. Most traditional practitioners are middle-aged women who are long-time residents of the village in which they practice. Common motivations are service and profit.

22.a. In Thailand and the Philippines over 90 percent of the traditional practitioners interviewed were female. In Bangladesh some men provide abortion services (Islam, 1982).

22.b. In Thailand practitioners averaged nearly 50 years of age; over one quarter had resided in their village for more than 11 years, and 42 percent had lived there since birth (Narkavonnakit, 1979). In the Philippines practitioners were 47 years old, on average, and over 60 percent had lived in their villages for over 20 years (Gallen, 1982).

Figure 3 Number of abortion-related deaths, by year, according to legal status of abortion, United States, 1965–85

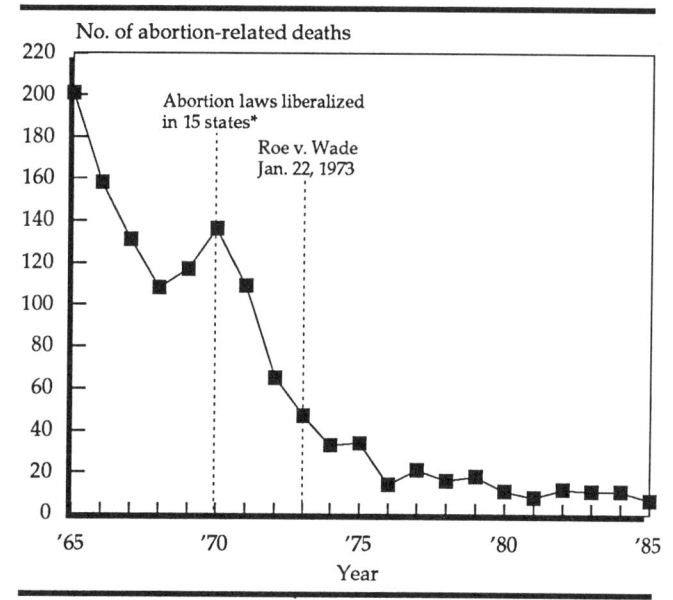

*By the end of 1970, 4 states had repealed their anti-abortion laws and 11 states had reformed them.
Note: Figure includes deaths from both legal and illegal abortions, but excludes spontaneous abortions.
Source: Gold, 1990, Figure 13, p. 27.
Reproduced with the permission of The Alan Guttmacher Institute from Rachel Benson Gold, *Abortion and Women's Health: A Turning Point for America*, 1990.

22.c. The educational level of practitioners reflects the availability of education within the country. In Bangladesh most traditional practitioners were illiterate (Islam, 1982). In the Philippines 17 percent had never been to school but 13 percent had completed graduate studies. In Thailand practitioners were evenly distributed among categories of no schooling, four years of schooling, and eight or more years of schooling (Narkavonnakit, 1979).

22.d. Traditional abortionists in the Philippines, Bangladesh, and Thailand offer their services in the belief that they meet a community need, as well as for income (Islam, 1982; Gallen, 1982; Narkavonnakit, 1979). In Bangladesh practitioners state that their acts save their clients' honor (the importance of performing acts that save honor is emphasized in the Muslim religion) (Islam, 1982).

23. Many traditional practitioners hesitate to perform abortions at gestations greater than four months. Most abortions appear to be performed early in the pregnancy. Practitioners may or may not provide medicines, follow-up service, and family planning advice or referral.

23.a. In the Philippines 75 percent of patients requested abortions during the first trimester of pregnancy, 80 percent took some form of medication afterwards, and over 50 percent of the women were told to return for a check-up after the procedure (Gallen, 1982).

23.b. In Thailand practitioners base their fees on the gestational age of the fetus. Over 50 percent of practitioners refused to perform abortions after three months of gestation, while two-thirds would not perform the procedure after four months. Half the practitioners routinely provided some kind of drug after the procedure, and one-third offered modern antibiotics (Narkavonnakit, 1979).

23.c. In the Philippines about half the abortion clients of traditional practitioners received advice about family planning (Gallen, 1982).

23.d. In Bangladesh some practitioners refused to perform abortions after the first trimester; others performed abortions in the third trimester, but refused women who had been pregnant for only one month. Some practitioners referred clients to menstrual regulation or sterilization clinics; others had never done so. Few practitioners treated complications of abortions, viewing such problems as being the patients' fault (Islam, 1982).

MODERN METHODS OF ABORTION

24.a. *Vacuum aspiration* is the safest widely available method of first-trimester abortion. It entails the removal of fetal tissue by vacuuming the uterus with either a manual or an electronic suction device (Liskin, 1980; Frejka et al., 1989; Henshaw, 1990). The cervix may or may not be dilated first, depending on its size and flexibility, the length of gestation, and the skill of the practitioner (IPAS, no date).

24.b. *Curettage*, common in countries where few surgeons are trained in suction methods, entails scraping the products of conception from the walls of the uterus. Risks of uterine perforation or incomplete abortion are greater with curettage than with suction methods (Henshaw, 1990).

24.c. *Menstrual regulation* (uterine evacuation without a pregnancy test) offers the option of guaranteeing subsequent nonpregnancy while leaving pregnancy status at the time of the procedure undetermined (Akhter, 1988; Dixon-Mueller, 1988). Nonpregnancy is guaranteed by evacuating the uterus using one of the methods described above.

24.d. *RU486*, in combination with a prostaglandin (PG) (taken orally), provides a safe and effective means of terminating pregnancies during the first eight or nine weeks after a missed period. It is over 95 percent effective up to 49 days after a missed period. Effectiveness declines slightly but significantly at durations of amenorrhea longer than 49 days (Ulmann, 1990). Some blood loss usually occurs with use of RU486/PG; in most cases blood flow is comparable to a normal period, lasting 1–16 days. In a trial of the method with 10,244 women, a blood transfusion was given in only .1 percent of the cases (Ulmann, 1990; Aubeny, 1990; Hill et al., 1990). In rare cases, RU486/PG has caused cardiac complications; therefore it is not used for women with various cardiovascular contraindications. It is also inappropriate for women with adrenal insufficiency or with the usual contraindications for prostaglandins (such as asthma or severe hypertension) (Klitsch, 1989). Contraindications related to age and smoking have also been debated (Ulmann, 1990). RU486/PG offers several advantages over other first-trimester methods of abortion: it is less invasive and requires less intervention than surgical methods; the decision of whether to use anesthesia is irrelevant; it is effective immediately after a missed period; and risks of laceration and perforation are nonexistent. However, access to competent medical services is important for treatment of complications, should they occur. With RU486/PG the woman takes more responsibility for implementing the method and ascertaining that a complete expulsion has occurred (Ulmann, 1990; Aubeny, 1990; Hill et al., 1990).

24.e. In the second trimester abortion is performed either by dilation and evacuation or by medical induction. The procedure chosen varies across countries and, within countries, across practitioners. Pregnancies of durations between 12 and 18 weeks are usually terminated by dilating the cervix and removing the products of conception with forceps (Henshaw, 1990). The uterus is then evacuated either by suction or by curettage. The procedure requires surgical expertise and can be stressful for medical personnel, but it is less traumatic for the woman than medical induction (Tietze and Henshaw, 1986). Pregnancies of durations longer than 18–20 weeks are terminated by medical induction (Henshaw, 1990). Uterine contractions are stimulated with oxytocin or prostaglandins. Saline solution is used when other agents are not available. Eventually the contractions expel the fetus. Medical induction is lengthier and riskier than other procedures (Tietze and Henshaw, 1986; Frejka et al., 1989).

NOTES

1. Data on national levels of abortion are very defective for developing countries, and statistics for developed countries are often incomplete. The relative frequency of abortion in different parts of the world is inferred from hospital data, surveys, and smaller area studies. Hospital data, while common, are rarely representative and always incomplete, as are data from family planning and health clinics. Abortion practitioners will sometimes describe their patients and methods, but it is unclear what populations they serve or how reliably they report on numbers of clients. In surveys and community-based studies women are asked about their experiences with abortion either directly or with the randomized response technique (RRT), which uses a physical device to allow interviewees to answer sensitive questions without the interviewer knowing their responses. Underreporting, however, is likely in all studies. Only 33 percent of Nigerian women who had received hospital treatment for complications of abortion admitted in interviews six months later to having undergone an abortion (Coeytaux, 1988). Questioning with the RRT yielded higher estimates of the incidence of abortion than did direct questioning in South Korea, Canada, Ethiopia, and Turkey; however, in South Korea, even with RRT, only 40 percent of women who were known to have had an abortion actually reported one (Tietze and Henshaw, 1986).

2. The *total abortion rate* is the number of abortions a woman would have during her lifetime if she experienced the current abortion rates at each age. *The abortion rate* is the number of abortions per 1,000 women of reproductive age. *The abortion ratio* is the number of abortions per live birth. An ideal ratio would relate abortions to pregnancies, but data on births are more easily obtained. One way to approximate the number of pregnancies is to add the number of births and abortions to an estimate of the number of spontaneous abortions and stillbirths; however, this is not generally done.

3. Because of underreporting, samples of women who admit experience with abortion are almost never representative of the true population of women who have had an abortion. Consequently, characteristics of women who choose abortions can be determined only tentatively.

4. Septic abortion is a condition in which either the endometrial cavity or its contents are infected. Septic abortion can occur when the uterus is not completely evacuated or when unclean instruments are used.

5. Deaths from complications of abortion are particularly likely to be underreported, because they are often classified as deaths from hemorrhage or infection (without noting that these conditions were caused by an abortion).

REFERENCES

Akhter, H. 1988. "Bangladesh." In *International Handbook on Abortion*, P. Sachdev, ed. New York: Glenwood Press. Pp. 36–48.

Anonymous. 1987. "Japan's fertility trends linked to late marriage, unique social factors, heavy reliance on abortion." *Family Planning Perspectives* 19(4):166–167.

Aubeny, E. 1990. "New perspective for patients: Drug induced abortion by RU486 and prostoglandins." Paper presented at the 1990 conference *From Abortion to Contraception*, Tbilisi, Georgia, 10–13 October.

Bulut, A. 1984. "Acceptance of effective contraceptive methods after induced abortion." *Studies in Family Planning* 15(6):281–284.

Castle, M.A., R. Likwa, and M. Whittaker. 1990. "Observations on abortion in Zambia." *Studies in Family Planning* 21(4):231–235.

Chaturachinda, K.S., S. Tangtrakul, S. Pongthai, and W. Phuapradit. 1981. "Abortion: An epidemiologic study at Ramithibodi Hospital, Bangkok." *Studies in Family Planning* 12(6/7):257–262.

Chhabra, S., N. Gupte, A. Mehta, and A. Sherde. 1988. "Medical termination of pregnancy and concurrent contraceptive adoption in rural India." *Studies in Family Planning* 4(19):244–247.

Coeytaux, F.M. 1988. "Induced abortion in sub-Saharan Africa: What we do and do not know." *Studies in Family Planning* 19(3):186–190.

Davis, K. 1963. "The theory of change and response in modern demographic history." *Population Index* 29:345–366.

Dixon-Mueller, R. 1988. "Innovations in reproductive health care: Menstrual regulation policies and programs in Bangladesh." *Studies in Family Planning* 19(3):129–140.

Flavier, J.M. and C.H.C. Chen. 1980. "Induced abortion in rural villages of Cavite, the Philippines: Knowledge, attitudes, and practice." *Studies in Family Planning* 11(2):65–71.

Fortney, J. 1981. "The use of hospital resources to treat incomplete abortions: Examples from Latin America." *Public Health Reports* 96(6):574–579.

Frejka, T. 1984. "Induced abortion and fertility: Selected aspects." *International Family Planning Perspectives* 11(4):125–129.

———.1993. "The role of induced abortion in contemporary fertility regulation." Paper presented at the General Conference of the IUSSP, 24 August-2 September.

Frejka, T. and L.C. Atkin. 1990. "The role of induced abortion in the fertility transition in Latin America." Paper presented at the Seminar on the Fertility Transition in Latin America, Buenos Aires 1990, IUSSP, Liège.

Frejka, T., L.C. Atkin, and O.L. Toro. 1989. "Research programs for the prevention of unsafe induced abortion and its adverse consequences in Latin America and the Caribbean." *Programs Division Working Paper*. Mexico City: The Population Council Regional Office for Latin America and the Caribbean.

Gallen, M. 1982. "Induced abortion in the Philippines: A study of clients and practitioners." *Studies in Family Planning* 13(2):35–44.

Gold, R. 1990. *Abortion and Women's Health: A Turning Point for America?* New York: Alan Guttmacher Institute.

Hakim-Elahi, E., H. Tovell, and M. Burnhill. 1990. "Complications of first-trimester abortion: A report of 170,000 cases." *Obstetrics and Gynecology* 76(1):129–135.

Henshaw, S. 1990. "Induced abortion: A world review, 1990." *Family Planning Perspectives* 22(2):76–89.

Hill, N., J. Ferguson, and I. MacKenzie. 1990. "The efficacy of oral mifepristone (RU 38,486) with a prostaglandin E_1 analog vaginal pessary for the termination of early pregnancy: Complications and patient acceptability." *The American Journal of Obstetrics and Gynecology* 162(2):414–417.

Hollerbach, P. and S. Diaz-Briquet. 1983. *Fertility Determinants in Cuba*. Report Number 26 of the Panel on Fertility Determinants. Washington, DC: National Academy Press.

IPAS (International Projects Assistance Service). No date. "Clinical guidelines for the use of manual vacuum aspiration in managing incomplete abortion." Carrboro, NC: IPAS.

Islam, S. 1982. "Case studies of indigenous abortion practitioners in rural Bangladesh." *Studies in Family Planning* 13(3):86–93.

Jacobson, J. 1990. "The global politics of abortion." *Worldwatch Paper* 97. Washington, DC: Worldwatch Institute.

Khan, A.R., S.F. Begum, D.L. Covington, B. Janowitz, S. James, and M. Potts. 1984. "Risks and costs of illegally induced abortion in Bangladesh." *Journal of Biosocial Sciences Supplement* 16(1):89–98.

Khan, M.E., B.C. Patel, and R. Chandrasekar. 1990. "A study of MTP acceptors and their subsequent contraceptive use." *Journal of Family Welfare* 36(3):70–85.

Klitsch, M. 1989. *RU-486: The Science and the Politics*. New York: Alan Guttmacher Institute.

Kwast, B.E. and J.A. Stevens. 1987. "Viral hepatitis as a major cause of maternal mortality in Addis Ababa, Ethiopia." *International Journal of Gynaecology and Obstetrics* 25:99–106.

Ladipo, O. 1989. "Preventing and managing complications of induced abortion in third world countries." *International Journal of Gynecology and Obstetrics* Supplement 3:21–28.

Leke, R.J. 1987. "Outcome of pregnancy and delivery at the Central Maternity Hospital, Yaoundé." *Annales Universitaires Sciences de la Santé* 4(1):322–330.

Liskin, L.S. 1980. "Complications of abortion in developing countries." *Population Reports* Series F, No. 7.

Mashabala, N. 1989. "Commentary on the causes and consequences of unwanted pregnancy from an African perspective." *International Journal of Gynecology and Obstetrics* Supplement 3:15–20.

Narkavonnakit, T. 1979. "Abortion in rural Thailand: A survey of practitioners." *Studies in Family Planning* 10(8/9):223–229.

Nnatu, S. 1988. "Nigeria." In *International Handbook on Abortion*. P. Sachdev, ed. New York: Glenwood Press.

Ovin, A., A. Orunsaye, M. Fall, and E. Asuquo. 1984. "Adolescent induced abortion in Benin City, Nigeria." *International Journal of Gynecology and Obstetrics* 19:10–15.

Potter, R.G. 1963. "Birth intervals: Structure and change." *Population Studies* 17:155–166.

Rochat, R., D. Kramer, P. Senanayake, and C. Howell. 1980. "Induced abortions and health problems in developing countries." *The Lancet* 11:484.

Royston, E. and S. Armstrong. 1989. *Preventing Maternal Deaths*. Geneva: World Health Organization.

Samil, R. 1989. "Commentary on menstrual regulation as a health service: Challenges in Indonesia." *International Journal of Gynecology and Obstetrics* Supplement 3:29–32.

Technical Working Group on "Meeting Women's Needs for Post-Abortion Family Planning." 1993. Bellagio, Italy. Proceedings and recommendations, forthcoming.

Tietze, C. 1964. "The demographic significance of legal abortion in Eastern Europe." *Demography* 1(1):119–125.

Tietze, C. and J. Bongaarts. 1975. "Fertility rates and abortion rates: Simulations of family limitation." *Studies in Family Planning* 6(5):114–120.

Tietze, C. and S. Henshaw. 1986. *Induced abortion: A world review*. 6th Edition. New York: The Alan Guttmacher Institute.

Toubia, N. 1989. "Measuring the rising costs of unwanted pregnancy in Khartoum, Sudan." In *Methodological Issues in Abortion Research*. F. Coeytaux, A. Leonard, and E. Royston, eds. New York: The Population Council.

Ulmann, A. 1990. "RU-486: Present and future uses." Paper presented at the 1990 conference, *From Abortion to Contraception*, Tbilisi, Georgia, 10–13 October.

World Health Organization (WHO). 1970. "Spontaneous and induced abortion." *Technical Report Series* No. 461. Geneva: WHO.

Wu, Z., E. Gao, X. Ku, M. Wang, W. Hong, and L. Chow. 1992. "Induced abortion among unmarried women in Shanghai, China." *Studies in Family Planning* 18(2):51–53.

Zatuchni, G.I. 1970. "Overview of program: Two-year experience." In *Post-partum Family Planning: A Report on the International Program*. G.I. Zatuchni, ed. New York: McGraw-Hill.

Chapter 10

CONTRACEPTION, FERTILITY PATTERNS, AND INFANT AND CHILD MORTALITY

1. **Contraceptive use acts to reduce infant and child mortality.**

   1.a. Contraceptive use lowers the number of births in a population. At constant mortality rates, fewer births mean fewer infant and child deaths. Fewer deaths lessen the strain on health care systems and increase the per-capita expenditure on health for any given level of funding, which may also act to reduce infant and child mortality (Bongaarts, 1987).

   1.b. Contraceptive use changes the distribution of births by reproductive parameters. Infant and child mortality rates will decline to the extent that fewer births in the new distribution occur to women with high-risk characteristics (Bongaarts, 1987; Trussell and Pebley, 1984; Winikoff, 1987; Potter, 1988).

   1.c. Contraceptive use may lower infant death rates by reducing unwanted births wherever those are selected for higher risk; moreover, some contraceptive methods protect the mother and thus the fetus or infant from sexually transmitted diseases (National Academy of Sciences, 1989).

   The above relationships are supported in subsequent sections, which rely upon the following types of evidence:

   * Bivariate relationships: the association of age, parity, and birth intervals with infant/child mortality
   * Multivariate relations: combinations of risk factors that affect infant/child mortality
   * Changes in the distribution of births as fertility declines
   * Changes in infant/child mortality from changes in the pace and ages at which childbearing occurs
   * Reduced infant/child mortality through prevention of unwanted births and sexually transmitted diseases.

BIVARIATE RELATIONSHIPS

Results presented below are from data from 25 countries where Demographic Health Surveys were conducted. The relationships for both infants and children are considered. The first year of life is treated as a whole, but note that patterns for neonates (babies under one month old) may be different from patterns for postneonates (babies 1–11 months old).

2. **Mortality rates typically exhibit a U-shaped curve with age and birth order. Mortality rates decline with increasing birth-interval lengths.**

Teenage Mothers

3. **Infants of teenagers experience higher mortality rates than do infants of women in their 20s.**

   3.a. In 23 of 25 developing countries (Ecuador and Botswana are the exceptions), infants of very young teenagers (below 17 years) fare worse than infants of older teenagers (17–19 years). Excess infant mortality associated with teenage births varies from under 10 percent (Sri Lanka and Bolivia) to over 60 percent (Zimbabwe and Paraguay). Mortality differentials for teen births diminish as children age.

Births to Older Women

4. **Mortality levels of infants born to women aged 30–39 are within 10 percent of the levels of infants born to women aged 20–29.**

   4.a. In 17 out of the 25 developing countries analyzed, this relationship holds true. In only two countries (Paraguay and Zimbabwe) do the excess risks of infants born to older mothers exceed 30 percent. For children, mortality patterns by age of the mother are less stable. In some countries children of older women do better than children of younger women; in other countries the reverse holds.

   4.b. In an Egyptian study the infant mortality rate for mothers aged 15–19 was 45 percent above that for mothers in their 20s (Ibrahim, 1993).

Birth Order

5. Infant mortality for first births is about 10 percent

above that for second- and third-order births.

5.a. Across 25 DHS countries infant mortality averages 76 per 1,000 live births for first births and 67 for second and third births; in only six countries is the order reversed. The mortality difference between first and second/third births decreases after infancy (see below).

6. **Risks associated with high-order births vary from region to region.**

6.a. In African countries infants of birth orders four to six do not appear to have higher mortality than do infants of orders two or three. In Latin America and Asia birth orders of four and higher are associated with excess infant mortality.

6.b. In the Egyptian study (see 4.b.) fifth and higher order births experienced 38 percent higher mortality than did those of the third and fourth order.

Preceding Interval Length

7. **Infants born after intervals shorter than two years have much higher mortality than do infants born after at least two years.**

7.a. In most DHS countries the excess mortality for short-interval births was 65 percent or greater. For children the results are less consistent, but risks generally are at least 15 percent higher for children born after short intervals (below two years), compared with children born after two- to four-year intervals.

The strong associations documented above are bivariate, which are not additive, since risk factors overlap:

* The presence of one risk factor often implies the presence of another. For example, births to teenagers are often either first births or poorly-spaced births.

* Additionally, socioeconomic status is often correlated both with infant and child mortality risks and with reproductive risk factors. For example, the relationship between birth order and infant and child mortality may be overstated if most children of birth orders higher than three are born to poor families, and controls for household income are not included.

* Survival status of a child's siblings influences both that child's mortality risks and the reproductive behavior of the child's mother. Mortality risks are higher for children whose siblings have died than for children whose siblings have survived. Risks of short birth intervals or high parity are higher for women whose children have died than for women whose children have survived because of biological and behavioral replacement mechanisms. Untangling risks associated with dead siblings from risks associated with short birth intervals or high parity is difficult.

* Duration of breastfeeding influences survival chances. Lengthier breastfeeding is associated with lower mortality risks and longer birth intervals. On the other hand, if a child dies, breastfeeding stops and conception may occur quickly, inducing a short birth interval.

MULTIVARIATE RELATIONSHIPS

8. **The effects of reproductive parameters on infant and child mortality persist (but are weakened) when controls for biodemographic and socioeconomic factors are introduced.**

Most of the results presented below come from a 34-country multivariate analysis of WFS data, with controls for a child's sex, birth order, interval length, and maternal education and age. These are drawn from Hobcraft (1987), unless otherwise noted.

Births to Teenagers

9. **On average, teenage births carry elevated risks.**

9.a. Children born to teenagers have 34 percent higher mortality before age five than do children born to mothers aged 25–34. Separate data for mothers below age 18 are revealing: Children born to women under age 18 have 42 percent higher mortality than do children born to women aged 25–34, while the excess mortality for children born to women aged 18–19 is only 13 percent.

9.b. The combination of a first birth with young maternal age is especially risky, producing excess mortality of 80 percent, in comparison with second- and third-order births of women 25–34.

Children of Older Women

10. **Evidence on the effects of childbearing among older women, independent of parity, is mixed.**

10.a. Children born to women over 35 do not suffer higher mortality than do those born to younger mothers, in the WFS analysis. In Indonesia and Pakistan children born to women over 35 actually have lower reported mortality than do children of younger women (controlling for birth order) (Martin et al., 1983). However, in Guatemala children of older women are at a significantly higher risk of mortality than children of younger women (controlling for birth order and spacing effects) (Pebley and Stupp, 1987).

First Births

11. **Infant mortality is higher for first births than for second and third births.**

    11.a. The infant mortality rate of first births averages 86 per 1,000, as compared with 53 per 1,000 for second and third births—a greater difference than that observed in the later DHS data (bivariate relationship) (see 5.a. above). The mortality difference between first- and higher-order births decreases after infancy, as seen in the child mortality rates.

    11.b. Levels of excess risk for firstborns vary substantially by country. In Indonesia, Sri Lanka, and parts of China, first births do not experience higher mortality, while in North Africa and the Middle East excess risks for firstborns are much higher than those in other regions (Martin et al., 1983; Trussell and Hammerslough, 1983; Tu, 1989).

Higher Order Births

12. **On average, the highest birth orders carry elevated risks.**

    12.a. Births of orders four, five, and six experience no excess mortality during infancy, but do experience 20 percent higher mortality during years one to five, compared with births of order two or three. Additionally, births of order 7+ face an under-five mortality risk that is 20 percent higher than that of births of order two or three.

Previous Birth Intervals

13. **Short birth intervals can carry an elevated risk for the child born second.**

    13.a. Children with a sibling who is close in age (less than two years older) face a 52 percent higher mortality risk than do children with siblings who are at least two years older. The effect is much larger for children whose closest older sibling was born less than two years before their own birthday but subsequently died.

    13.b. In Bangladesh and the Philippines children born within 15 months of a preceding birth are 60–80 percent more likely to die before age two than are other children, even after controlling for prematurity. In Bangladesh the harmful effects of a short preceding birth interval are confined to the first month of life (Koenig et al., 1990).

    13.c. Mortality risks for children with a sibling who is close in age appear to be substantially higher in North Africa and the Middle East than in other regions. Closely spaced births are common in these areas.

Subsequent Birth Intervals

14. **Short birth intervals can carry an elevated risk for the child born first.**

    14.a. Children with a sibling born within 12 months after their own birth have a mortality risk between the ages of one and five that is 77 percent higher than that of children whose next youngest sibling is at least two years younger. A birth 12–18 months after the index child's birth raises its mortality risk by 48 percent. A pregnancy of duration three months or more by a child's second birthday raises the child's mortality risk between ages one and five by 55 percent.

Combinations of Risk Factors

Hobcraft (1991) analyzes the effects of various family formation patterns on mortality below age five, using data from 18 developing countries in which Demographic and Health Surveys were conducted. He divides births into 10 categories based on the mother's age and parity, the length of her preceding birth interval, and her prior pace of fertility.

Risk categories are defined as follows:

* Age: Teenage births and births to women aged 20–34 (numbers of women over 35 were inadequate for analysis)

* Birth order: First births and later births

* Spacing: Well-spaced births (after intervals of 2+ years) and poorly spaced births (intervals of less than 2 years)

* Pace of reproduction: (for women aged 20–34). Hobcraft categorizes the pace of reproduction as

slow, medium, or fast, based on the number of children by age of mother, as shown below.

Pace of childbearing, according to number of children and mother's age

Pace	Age 20–24	Age 25–29	Age 30–34
Slow	2	2–3	2–4
Medium	3	4–5	5–6
Fast	4+	6+	7+

These categories give rise to the following 10 risk categories:

Births to teenagers: (1) First births; (2) poorly-spaced later births; (3) well-spaced later births.

Births to women 20–34: (4) First births.

Later births: (5) Poorly-spaced births, slow pace; (6) poorly-spaced births, medium pace; (7) poorly-spaced births, fast pace; (8) well-spaced births, slow pace; (9) well-spaced births, medium pace; (10) well-spaced births, fast pace.

15. **Risks of children born to women aged 20 to 34 vary according to the combination of birth order, prior pace of reproduction, and the length of the preceding interval.**

15.a. First births to women aged 30–34 have a 6 percent higher mortality than do higher order, well-spaced births, but differentials for first births vary substantially by country. First births in Kenya, Mali, and Tunisia face higher risks than first births in other countries (excess mortality of about 30 percent), while first births in Peru, Colombia, and the Dominican Republic have lower mortality rates than do higher order births.

15.b. Compared to children born at a medium pace, those born at a slow pace have 8 percent lower mortality and those born at a fast pace have 24 percent higher mortality (all with reference to well-spaced, higher order births to women aged 20–34). Mortality differentials by the pace of reproduction are larger in Brazil, Colombia, Ecuador, and Peru than in other countries.

15.c. Poorly-spaced births have high excess mortality risks compared with well-spaced births; the size of the difference in risk increases with the prior pace of fertility. Relative to all well-spaced children, poorly-spaced children suffer elevated mortality: 35 percent higher if born at a slow pace, 80 percent higher if born at a medium pace, and even 123 percent higher if born at a fast pace.

16. **Children of teenage mothers experience higher mortality, compared with well-spaced births to women 20–34, regardless of birth order or spacing.**

16.a. First births to teenage women have 46 percent excess risk compared with well-spaced births to women 20–34.

16.b. Higher-order births to teenagers have an excess mortality of 35 percent when they are well-spaced, 117 percent when they are poorly-spaced.

CHANGES IN THE DISTRIBUTION OF BIRTHS AS FERTILITY DECLINES

17. **Contraceptive use acts to reduce fertility, and as fertility falls the proportion of all births that are first births tends to rise, while the proportion of births at order five or higher tends to fall. This change in the composition of births implies a change in the infant mortality rate, because different subgroups have different mortality rates. The change may or may not reduce the infant mortality rate, although in absolute terms fewer births certainly mean fewer infant and child deaths.**

17.a. The proportion of first births has risen in each of eight countries where both WFS and DHS data are available. The largest increases in first births occurred in countries where fertility has declined dramatically, such as Thailand, Colombia, Sri Lanka, and Trinidad and Tobago (Hobcraft, 1991).

17.b. The proportion of fifth and later births decreased in 11 countries where fertility declined significantly between the 1960s and the 1970s–80s. In the 1960s the proportions ranged from .23 to .45. In the following decades the range was from .02 to .22 (National Academy of Sciences, 1989).

18. **As fertility declines, the proportion of births to older women generally declines, while the direction of change for the proportion of births to younger women is mixed.**

18.a. In the 11 countries mentioned above the proportion of births to older women declined in all countries. The proportion of births to younger women increased in only six countries. In four countries the proportion of births to young women decreased, and in one country the proportion remained the same (National Academy of Sciences, 1989).

19. **It is unclear how the distribution of births changes**

by preceding interval length as fertility declines.

19.a. As fertility fell, the proportion of births occurring at short intervals decreased as well, in eight of 10 countries for which data were available (National Academy of Sciences, 1989).

19.b. In Thailand, Colombia, Sri Lanka, and Trinidad and Tobago, the proportion of poorly-spaced births has declined with decreases in fertility levels (Hobcraft, 1991).

19.c. However, cross-sectional analyses often show that countries with lower fertility rates have a higher proportion of births at short intervals than do countries with higher fertility rates (Hobcraft, 1987; Bongaarts, 1987; Trussell, 1988). Also, in Korea, where fertility declined dramatically in the 1960s, the proportion of women giving birth to a second child within two years of the first increased from 35 percent in 1960 to almost 50 percent in 1970 (Ross and Madhavan, 1981; Rindfuss et al., 1982)

CHANGES IN INFANT AND CHILD MORTALITY RATES DUE TO CHANGES IN THE PACE AND AGES AT WHICH CHILDBEARING OCCURS

20. Changes in family formation patterns have the potential to substantially alter the mortality experience of individual families.

20.a. In a six-child family, children born to women who begin childbearing at age 22 and space births at three-year intervals are less than half as likely to die before age two as children whose mothers begin childbearing at age 18 and space births at 18-month intervals (Hobcraft, 1987).

20.b. Most women who begin childbearing early and reproduce quickly will have a child die, while less than half of the women who delay childbearing and reproduce slowly will have a child die (Hobcraft, 1987).

20.c. One quarter of women with poor reproductive patterns will experience the death of two children under age two. Only 8 percent of women with better reproductive patterns can expect two children to die (Hobcraft, 1987).

21. Changes in family formation patterns have the potential to alter overall mortality rates within countries.

21.a. If teenagers delayed all births until they were 20 and stopped reproducing by age 34, gains in child survival would range up to 12 percent. (However, results are from DHS data, which are based on the strong assumption that all excess mortality for teenage mothers would disappear if they delayed childbearing).

21.b. In Peru an increase in birth intervals to at least 18 months would reduce the risk of death during the first year of life and in the next four years by 13 percent and 9 percent, respectively. Eliminating later conceptions occurring before the child was 3, 6, or 9 months old would lower mortality by 4 percent to 11 percent (Palloni and Tienda, 1986).

21.c. In Pakistan postneonatal mortality would decline by 14 percent if all birth intervals shorter than 24 months increased to 24–29 months (Cleland and Sathar, 1984).

22. Changes in the distribution of births by reproductive parameters have contributed to declines in infant and childhood mortality.

22.a. Favorable changes in the distribution of births across risk categories have contributed to declines in mortality below age five, in seven of eight developing countries from which WFS and DHS data are available. (Relative risk patterns have worsened, however, offsetting some gains) (Hobcraft, 1991).[1]

22.b. In Costa Rica and Trinidad and Tobago changes in the distribution of births over a 10-year period (1–5 years before the WFS survey versus 11–16 years before the survey) accounted for about a 15 percent decline in mortality rates between the two periods. The benefits of the distributional change in births were smaller in other countries, but they often accounted for around 20 percent of the decline in mortality between the two periods (Hobcraft, 1987).[2]

REDUCED INFANT/CHILD MORTALITY THROUGH PREVENTION OF UNWANTED BIRTHS AND SEXUALLY TRANSMITTED DISEASES

23. Contraceptive use reduces the number of unwanted children, thereby reducing infant and child mortality.

23.a. Unwanted children probably experience elevated mortality rates. In Matlab, Bangladesh, as contraceptive prevalence increased from below 10 percent to 34 percent, the mortality rates of girls 2–4 years of age decreased significantly. No change occurred in the mortality rate of boys that age. A multivariate analysis of time-series data shows the inverse association between contraceptive use and female child mortality to be significant (Phillips et al., 1987).

23.b. Preventing the birth of unwanted children through contraceptive use (or abortion) will prevent some infant deaths and may lower the infant mortality *rate*. Unwanted children may die more frequently than wanted children, either because they are born disproportionately to high-risk women (Potter, 1988) or because their families do not or cannot care for them properly (National Academy of Sciences, 1989).

24. Barrier contraceptives protect infant health and survival by impairing the transmission of sexually transmitted diseases (STDs).

24.a. Barrier methods of contraception may protect women from herpes simplex and cytomegalovirus (CMV), which have been linked with fetal death, intrauterine growth retardation, prematurity, malformations, congenital infection, and various postnatal infections. Hepatitis B in pregnant women is associated with prematurity and neonatal and postneonatal infections (National Academy of Sciences, 1989).

24.b. Barrier methods of contraception protect women from contracting infections that they could transmit to their children during gestation or through breastmilk (National Academy of Sciences, 1989).

24.c. Wasserheit (1989) concludes that STDs "...are common in almost all of the developing countries in which they have been investigated..." (p. 153). Examining over 60 studies, she found that 10–25 percent of women in various subgroups had gonococcal cervicitis (with some results both below and above that range) and a somewhat higher percent had vaginitis. (Most subgroups came from clinical settings: antenatal, family planning, peripartum, as well as gynecology and STD clinics; a few studies were on a population basis). STD levels are higher in sub-Saharan Africa than in other regions.

Wasserheit notes that "...the population pyramid is heavily weighted with individuals in the age groups of most intense sexual activity" and that family planning programs may experience elevated termination rates because women confuse their STD symptoms with side effects from their contraceptive method. Moreover, contraceptive acceptance rates may suffer because women fear that their STD will impair their fertility. She calls for the addition of STD screening and treatment in all related reproductive health services.

Evidence from both developed and developing countries indicates that the HIV virus can be transmitted across the placental membrane and during delivery through contact with infected maternal blood (Senturia and Peckam, 1987). Children born to mothers infected with HIV have a 25–35 percent risk of HIV infection (Ellerbrock et al., 1991). Additionally, HIV virus has been identified in children delivered to women who were seronegative at the time of delivery but in whom HIV was later isolated. This finding suggests that breastfeeding is a mode of transmission from mother to child (Ziegler et al., 1985; Lepage et al., 1987). The AIDS virus has been isolated in breastmilk (Thiry et al., 1985).

NOTES

1. Hobcraft calculates mortality rates for children under five from both the DHS and the WFS data. He decomposes differences in rates into portions due to (1) a change in the baseline, or reference risk group (well-spaced births to women aged 20–34, (2) changes in the distribution of births across risk categories, and (3) changes in the relative mortality of births in different risk categories.

2. Hobcraft examines fertility patterns and mortality levels in WFS countries 11–16 years before the survey and 1–5 years before the survey. He decomposes changes in mortality rates between the two periods into portions that result from a change in the level of risk and those that result from a change in the distribution of births.

REFERENCES

Bongaarts, J. 1987. "Does family planning reduce mortality rates?" *Population and Development Review* 13(2):323–334.

Cleland, J. and Z. Sathar. 1984. "The effect of birth spacing on childhood mortality in Pakistan." *Population Studies* 38(3):401–418.

Ellerbrock, T., T. Bush, M. Chamberland, and M. Oxtoby. 1991. "Epidemiology of women with AIDS in the United States, 1981 through 1990." *Journal of the American Medical Association* 265(22):2,971–2,975.

Hobcraft, J. 1987. "Does family planning save children's lives?" Technical Background Paper prepared for the International Conference on Better Health for Women and Children Through Family Planning, Nairobi, Kenya, October.

Hobcraft, J. 1991. "Child Spacing and Child Mortality." *Demographic and Health Surveys World Conference Proceedings*, Vol.2:1,157–1,181. Columbia, Maryland: IRD/Macro International.

Ibrahim, B. 1993. Personal communication, based upon *Maternal Health and Infant Mortality in Egypt*. Cairo: Central Agency for Public Mobilization and Statistics and UNICEF.

Koenig, M., J. Phillips, O. Campbell, and S. D'Souza. 1990. "Birth intervals and childhood mortality in rural Bangladesh." *Demography* 27(2):251–265.

Lepage, P., P. Van de Perre, M. Carael, F. Nsengumuremyi, J. Nkurunziza, J. Butzler, and S. Sprecher. 1987. "Postnatal transmission of HIV from mother to child." *The Lancet* August, 15: 400.

Martin, L., J. Trussell, F. Salvail, and N. Shah. 1983. "Covariates of child mortality in the Philippines, Indonesia, and Pakistan: An analysis based on hazard models." *Population Studies* 37:417–433.

National Academy of Sciences. 1989. *Contraception and Reproduction: Health Consequences for Women and Children in the Developing World.* Report by the Working Group on the Health Consequences of Contraceptive Use and Controlled Fertility. Washington, DC: National Academy Press.

Palloni, A. and M. Tienda. 1986. "The effects of breastfeeding and pace of childbearing on mortality at early ages." *Demography* 23(1): 31–52.

Pebley, A. and P.W. Stupp. 1987. "Reproductive patterns and child mortality in Guatemala." *Demography* 24(1):43–60.

Phillips, J., T. Legrand, M. Koenig, and J. Chakraborty. 1987. "The impact of a maternal and child health experiment on infant and child mortality in Matlab, Bangladesh." Paper prepared for the annual meeting of the Population Association of America, Chicago, April 30–May 2.

Potter, J. 1988. "Does family planning reduce infant mortality? Comment." *Population and Development Review* 14(1):179–187.

Rindfuss, R., L. Bumpass, J. Palmore, and Dae Woo Han. 1982. "The transformation of Korean child-spacing practices." *Population Studies* 36(1):87–104.

Ross, J. and S. Madhavan. 1981. "A Gompertz model for birth interval analysis." *Population Studies* 35(3):439–454.

Senturia, Y.D. and C.S. Peckam. 1987. "HIV infection in children: Sizing up the paediatric problem." *Paediatric Perinatal Epidemiology* 1(2):143–51.

Thiry, L., S. Sprecher-Goldberger, T. Jonkheer, J. Levy, P. Van de Perre, P. Henrivaux, J. Cogniaux-Le Clerc, and N. Clumeck. 1985. "Isolation of AIDS virus from cell-free breastmilk of three healthy virus carriers." *The Lancet* October 19:890–891.

Trussell, J. 1988. "Does family planning reduce infant mortality? An exchange." *Population and Development Review* 14(1):171–178.

Trussell, J. and C. Hammerslough. 1983. "A hazards-model analysis of the covariates of infant and child mortality in Sri Lanka." *Demography* 20(1):1–26.

Trussell, J. and A. Pebley. 1984. "The potential impact of changes in fertility on infant, child, and maternal mortality." *Studies in Family Planning* 15(6):267–280.

Tu, Ping. 1989. "The effects of breastfeeding and birth spacing on child survival in China." *Studies in Family Planning* 20(6):332–342.

Wasserheit, Judith N. 1989. "The significance and scope of reproductive tract infections among third world women." *International Journal of Gynaecology and Obstetrics* Suppl. 3:145–168.

Winikoff, B. 1987. "Family planning and the health of women and children." *Technology in Society* 9:415–438.

Ziegler, J., D. Cooper, R. Johnson, and J. Gold. 1985. "Postnatal transmission of AIDS-associated retrovirus from mother to infant." *The Lancet* April 20:896–897.

Chapter 11

CONTRACEPTIVE USE AND MATERNAL MORBIDITY/MORTALITY

Complications from pregnancy and childbirth can cause illness, injury, or death. Contraceptive use benefits women's health by reducing the absolute number of pregnancies, by reducing septic abortions, and by helping to restrict childbearing to those ages and parities for which risks of obstetric complications are smallest (ages 20 to 34 and low parities).

DATA AND MEASUREMENT

1. Maternal mortality is defined as the death of a woman while she is pregnant or within 42 days of a pregnancy termination. Direct deaths result from complications of pregnancy or labor. Indirect deaths result from diseases that pregnancy aggravates, such as hepatitis or malaria.

    1.a. The *maternal mortality ratio*, the number of maternal deaths per 100,000 live births, measures the level of obstetric risk associated with pregnancy and can be combined with the total fertility rate to estimate a woman's lifetime chance of dying from pregnancy-related causes (Blacker, 1987).

    1.b. The *maternal mortality rate*, the number of maternal deaths per 100,000 women of reproductive age, reflects both the medical risks of pregnancy and the level of fertility within a population. The maternal mortality rate indicates the relative importance of maternal mortality as a cause of death when compared with other causes or with the overall death rate for women of reproductive age.

2. Measuring maternal mortality is difficult. The number of maternal deaths is small relative to the number of women exposed to the risk, so reliable measures require large samples (Winikoff, 1987). Vital registration systems and retrospective samples may undercount both deaths and live births (Zimicki, 1989). The pregnancy status of a woman who dies may go unreported.

    2.a. Hospital-based studies compare the number of maternal deaths in the hospital to the number of live births in the hospital over some time period. These data are unrepresentative in developing countries, because only a select subset of women give birth in hospitals, and those who do are rarely followed for 42 days (Adetoro, 1987; Trussell and Pebley, 1984). Prospective population-based studies are more representative but rare (Zimicki, 1989). Recently, researchers have interviewed women as to whether their sisters died from causes related to pregnancy. Preliminary evidence from The Gambia, Sudan, Bolivia, and Egypt indicates that this method yields plausible estimates (Graham et al., 1989; Rutenberg and Sullivan, 1991). Brothers may also be interviewed about their sisters (Graham et al., 1990.)

EXTENT OF MATERNAL MORTALITY AND MORBIDITY

Maternal Mortality

3. Maternal mortality claims the lives of hundreds of thousands of women of reproductive age each year. Most of these women live in the developing world.

    3.a. In 1988 an estimated 509,000 women, 99 percent of them from developing countries, died from causes related to pregnancy and childbirth (see *Table 1*) (World Health Organization, 1991).[1]

    3.b. More maternal deaths occur in India in one week than in all of Europe in an entire year (Royston and Lopez, 1987). One woman in every 21 in Africa will die of complications of pregnancy or delivery. In Northern Europe, only one woman in every 9,850 will die (Maine, no date).

    3.c. By recent WHO estimates, Africa is the region with the highest number (630) of maternal deaths per 100,000 live births. The ratio in Asia is 380 per 100,000, and it is 200 per 100,000 in Latin America and the Caribbean. For developed countries the average ratio is around 26 per 100,000 (WHO, 1991).

    3.d. Maternal mortality ratios across 12 subregions of the developing world range widely, from 120 to 760 per 100,000 live births as of 1988 (see *Table 1*). By far the highest rates occur in sub-Saharan Africa.

    3.e. If women in all countries faced the same risks

when pregnant as do women in the developed world, 460,000 fewer women would die each year (Royston and Lopez, 1987).

4. **Children suffer greatly when their mothers die. Each woman who dies from pregnancy-related causes leaves behind more than one child, on average (Winikoff, 1987).**

4.a. In Matlab (1960s) 95 percent of infants whose mothers died in childbirth died within a year (Chen et al., 1974). Between 1976 and 1985, three quarters of the children born to women who died from pregnancy-related causes also died within a year (Koenig et al., 1988).

4.b. In a rural area of The Gambia pregnant women were followed between 1982 and 1983. Live births accompanied eight of 15 maternal deaths. All of these children died in infancy (Greenwood et al., 1987).

Morbidity

5. **For each woman who dies from pregnancy-related causes, many others experience disabling injuries and infections.**

5.a. In Colombia, Pakistan, Syria, and the Philippines, 3–25 percent of women under age 45 suffered from uterine prolapse, a painful condition where the uterus descends into the vagina (Lettenmaier et al., 1988).

5.b. In parts of Africa many women suffer from openings between the vagina and urinary tract that cause incontinence. The condition is especially prevalent among teenagers and women experiencing obstructed labor or female circumcision. Often these women become social outcasts (Harrison, 1987; Starrs, 1987; Tahzib, 1983).

5.c. In Nigerian and Kenyan studies 8–20 percent of women developed genital tract infections after delivery. Such infections increase the chance of contracting pelvic inflammatory disease, having an ectopic pregnancy[2], or becoming infertile (Lettenmaier et al., 1988).

6. **Though pregnancy and childbearing make extra nutritional demands on women, little evidence so far supports the theory that frequent or rapid childbearing harms a mother's nutritional status.**

6.a. Neither a woman's hemoglobin levels nor her ponderal index (weight squared, divided by height) were associated with age, parity, or birth-interval length in a multinational study conducted by the World Health Organization (reviewed in Winikoff and Castle, 1988).

6.b. No relationship between length of time spent pregnant or breastfeeding and cumulative nutritional status emerged from a study of Ugandan women (Costello, 1986).

6.c. Many studies rely on simple measures of childbearing patterns and nutritional status, so the lack of an empirical relationship thus far should not be taken as conclusive evidence that one does not exist (Merchant and Martorell, 1988).

CAUSES OF MATERNAL MORTALITY
Direct Causes

7. Hemorrhage, eclampsia, obstructed labor, infection, and complications from induced abortion are the major causes of maternal mortality.[3]

Table 1 Estimates of maternal mortality and numbers of live births, by region, ca. 1983 and 1988, developing and developed countries

Region	Maternal mortality ratio (per 100,000 live births)[a] 1983	1988	Live births (millions) 1983[b]	1988[b]	Maternal deaths (000s)[a] 1983	1988
World	390	370	128.3	137.6	500	509
Developed countries	30	26	18.2	17.3	6	4
Developing countries	450	420	110.1	120.3	494	505
Africa	640	630	23.4	26.7	150	169
Northern	500	360	4.8	4.9	24	18
Western	700	760	7.6	8.7	54	66
Eastern	660	680	7.0	8.8	46	60
Middle	690	710	2.6	3.0	18	21
Southern	570	270	1.4	1.3	8	4
Asia	420	380	73.9	81.2	308	310
Western	340	280	4.1	4.4	14	12
Southern	650	570	35.6	39.6	230	224
Southeastern	420	340	12.4	12.5	52	42
Eastern	55	120	21.8	24.6	12	32
Latin America/Caribbean	270	200	12.6	12.2	34	25
Central	240	160	3.7	3.5	9	6
Caribbean	220	260	0.9	0.8	2	2
South	290	220	8.0	8.0	23	17
Northern America	12	12	4.0	4.0	1	1
Europe	27	23	6.6	6.4	2	1
Oceania	300	600	0.2	0.2	2	1
USSR	50	45	5.2	5.2	3	2

[a] World Health Organization estimates.
[b] Estimates for 1980–85 from *United Nations Demographic Indicators of Countries: Estimates and Projections as Assessed in 1980*. United Nations, Department of International Economic and Social Affairs, New York, 1982.
[c] Estimates for 1985–90 from *United Nations Demographic Indicators of Countries: Estimates and Projections as Assessed in 1990*. United Nations, Department of International Economic and Social Affairs, New York, 1991.
Source: World Health Organization (WHO). 1991. *Weekly Epidemiological Record* No. 47, 22 November. Table 1, p. 346.

7.a. Hemorrhage and complications of induced abortion accounted for almost 40 percent of maternal deaths in Matlab, Bangladesh between 1976 and 1985. Eclampsia, infection, and obstructed labor led to most of the other deaths (Fauveau et al., 1988).

7.b. In Lusaka, Zambia 20 percent of maternal deaths resulted from eclampsia. Complications of abortion killed almost 17 percent of the women. Infection, hemorrhage, and complications of infectious diseases were also major causes of maternal mortality (Mhango et al., 1986).

7.c. In Jamaica eclampsia, hemorrhage, ectopic pregnancy, and abortion accounted for two-thirds of maternal deaths (Walker et al., 1985, cited in Zimicki, 1989).

Indirect Causes

8. **Hepatitis, anemia, and malaria are the most common indirect causes of maternal mortality. About 25 percent of maternal deaths are from indirect causes.**

8.a. Viral hepatitis is one of the six major causes of maternal death in Ethiopia, Nigeria, Ghana, Malawi, and South Africa (Kwast and Stevens, 1987), and is also an important contributor to maternal death in China and India (Lettenmaier et al., 1988).

8.b. Parasite activity associated with endemic malaria is heavier and more frequent during a woman's first and second pregnancies than when she is not pregnant, which increases the risk of anemia (Zimicki, 1989; Lettenmaier et al., 1988).

8.c. In 12 Indonesian hospitals anemic women died during childbirth four times more frequently than did nonanemic women. Similar results are reported from Malaysia (Lettenmaier et al., 1988). Anemia worsens the deleterious effects of blood loss and can contribute to heart failure (Zimicki, 1989).

8.d. Pregnancy can ignite inactive tuberculosis — an indirect cause of mortality in some areas (Lettenmaier et al., 1988; Maine et al., 1985).

REPRODUCTIVE RISK FACTORS
Age

9. **Women below age 20 and over age 30 die more frequently during pregnancy and childbearing than do women in their 20s.**

9.a. In Matlab, Bangladesh maternal mortality ratios for women under age 15 were five times higher and ratios for older teen mothers were two times higher than those for women aged 20–24 (Chen et al., 1974; Koenig et al., 1988). Similar patterns hold in Zaria, Nigeria (Harrison and Rossiter, 1985).

9.b. Younger women are especially likely to suffer from pre-eclampsia and eclampsia, obstructed labor, and malaria (Zimicki, 1989).

9.c. In Nigeria women over age 30 face a 2.5 times greater risk of dying per pregnancy than do women 20–24 (Royston and Lopez, 1987). In Bangladesh women over 30 die much more frequently from pregnancy-related causes than do women 20–24 (Chen et al., 1974; Koenig et al., 1988). Similarly, Jamaican women aged 40–44 experience risks five times higher than women who are 20 years younger (Royston and Lopez, 1987).

Parity/Gravidity

10. **Women pregnant for the first time and women pregnant for the fifth time or more die more frequently from pregnancy-related causes than do other women.**

10.a. Women pregnant for the first time faced higher risks of death than did women of higher parities in all of the population-based studies and most of the hospital-based studies reviewed by Zimicki (1989). Eclampsia is the most frequent cause of death for these women. Women having their first child in Matlab, Bangladesh had over three times the risk of death of women having their third child (1976–85) (Koenig et al., 1988).

10.b. Women of parity five and above have 1.5 to 3 times the risk of death of women at parity two or three (National Academy of Sciences, 1989). Fetuses of women of high parity often lie in awkward positions, complicating delivery (Zimicki, 1989). High-parity women are more likely to require blood transfusions during delivery and to die of hemorrhage (Rinehart et al., 1984). In Matlab, Bangladesh maternal mortality ratios for women of parity six or higher were three times higher than were those for women of parity two (Chen et al., 1974).

10.c. The J-shaped relationship between parity and maternal mortality ratios holds across countries with different levels of mortality and socioeconomic development (Zimicki, 1989; Winikoff and Sullivan,

1987). Generally, however, as conditions within a country improve, the curve becomes flatter (National Academy of Sciences, 1989).

Combination of Age and Parity

11. **Age and parity are closely related. Efforts to separate their effects on maternal mortality risks have yielded mixed results.**[4]

   11.a. In hospital-based studies the relationship between parity and risk of death or complications is stronger than that for age. Within age groups risks rise with parity, but within parity groups risks are often constant by age (Zimicki, 1989).

   11.b. Data from Matlab for the late 1960s indicate that for women at the extremes of both age and parity (young age-low parity or old age-high parity), increments in either age or parity are important. For women in the middle ranges, on the other hand, an incremental change in age or parity does not substantially change risks (Zimicki, 1989).

   11.c. However, data from Matlab for the 1970s and 1980s lead to a different conclusion. At each parity older women face higher risks than do younger women, while high parity carries a higher risk only for the oldest ages (Koenig et al., 1988).

Birth Intervals

12. **Almost nothing is known about the relationship between short birth intervals and maternal mortality. No studies specifically address this question (Zimicki, 1989; National Academy of Sciences, 1989; Winikoff, 1987).**

INTERVENTIONS

In developed countries maternal risks to women today are only one to two percent of their levels 100 years ago (Rochat, 1981). Moreover, between 1983 and 1988 maternal mortality ratios declined from about 420 to 380 deaths per 100,000 live births in Asia, and from about 270 to 200 per 100,000 in Latin America. The improvements point to the potential for gains in decreasing maternal mortality.

Among other measures, such as increasing the availability of prenatal care and medical attendance at delivery, increasing the use of contraceptives is an appealing means of reducing the absolute numbers of maternal deaths. By preventing pregnancies, contraceptive use avoids both abortions and births and the associated risks altogether (apart from contraceptive failure). Numbers and rates of maternal deaths will fall at least in proportion to the reductions in pregnancies and births.[5]

13. **Contraceptive use can reduce maternal mortality very substantially by decreasing the aggregate number of births and the number of births per woman.**

   13.a. If women who say that they want no more children actually have no more children, the number of births would decline by an average of 17 percent in Africa, 33 percent in Asia, and 35 percent in Latin America. The number of maternal deaths should fall by at least as much (WFS data, reported in Royston and Lopez, 1987).

   13.b. In Matlab, Bangladesh maternal mortality rates in two areas diverged significantly as contraceptive prevalence increased sharply in one area but not in the other. In the treatment area contraceptive prevalence rose from 8 percent in 1975 to 44 percent in 1985. In the control area prevalence rose from 8 percent in 1975 to only 16 percent in 1984. Before 1978 maternal mortality rates in the two areas were similar, but from 1978–85 the rate in the treatment area was only 66 per 100,000 women, while that in the control area was 121 per 100,000 women (a statistically significant difference). The maternal mortality ratios (deaths per 100,000 live births) were not significantly different in the two areas. Thus, contraceptive use helped to reduce the number and rate of women who died, even though it did not reduce the risk of death per pregnancy.

   13.c. The lifetime risk of maternal mortality decreases when women have fewer children, even if the risk per pregnancy is constant. Childbearing in Bali is four times more risky than it is in Egypt; however, Balinese fertility is much lower than Egyptian fertility, so Balinese women are only 1.5 times more likely to die from maternity-related causes than are their Egyptian counterparts (Fortney, 1988).

14. **Use of contraceptives, by preventing unwanted pregnancies, can lower the number of unsafe abortions.**

   14.a. Unwanted pregnancies end in abortion more often than do wanted pregnancies. Prevention of unwanted pregnancies through the use of contraceptives can reduce mortality from complications of abortions, particularly if abortions are unsafe or illegal. Contraceptive use by Chilean women increased from 3 percent in 1964 to 23 percent in 1978. During the same period the number of women hospitalized for complications of abortion decreased by 33 percent, and the number of deaths from abortion plummeted (Rinehart et al., 1984; Maine, no date).

14.b. Unwanted pregnancies and abortions often occur to high-risk women (Rinehart et al., 1984). In South Africa 46 percent of women dying from complications of abortion were of parity five or higher, and 60 percent were unmarried (Barford and Parkes, 1977).

15. **Use of contraceptives can change the distribution of pregnancies and births so that proportionately fewer occur to very young women, older women, and women of high parity. Most pregnancies and births, however, do not fall into high-risk categories, so the effect of a distributional change on the overall maternal mortality ratio is attenuated.**

15.a. Most births and deaths occur to women in "safe" categories of age and parity, which limits the extent to which the maternal mortality ratio will fall through changes in the distribution of births by age and parity. A strategy that focuses only on high-risk women will ignore one-half to two-thirds of the women who will die (Winikoff, 1987).

15.b. Strategies to prevent maternal deaths by focusing on high-risk groups are further limited, since some members of those groups actively want more children or will not use contraceptives. A more feasible and effective strategy is to focus broadly on couples who want no more children (soon or ever), since those numbers are large. Unwanted pregnancies lead disproportionately to unsafe abortions, and in any case unwanted births fall heavily in the upper age and higher parity groups (Maine, 1988; Rooks and Winikoff, 1990).

15.c. Achieving large reductions in maternal mortality by focusing only on high-risk groups may require preventing a large proportion of all births. For example, in Bangladesh in the 1960s, eliminating births to women under age 20 or above parity four would have lowered maternal mortality by 58 percent but would have required preventing 43 percent of all births (Winikoff and Sullivan, 1987).

15.d. Additionally, the potential for lowering the maternal mortality *ratio* by eliminating high-parity births is reduced by the rise in the proportion of first births as the other births are prevented (Winikoff, 1987; Blacker, 1987); this is especially true if the safer, middle-parity births also decline.

15.e. In Matlab Bangladesh, maternal mortality ratios were not reduced significantly in an area in which contraceptive prevalence rose to 44 percent, in comparison with an area where contraceptive prevalence remained below 20 percent. Maternal mortality ratios did not change because many of the shifts in the distribution of childbearing were among groups with similar risks (ages 20–34, parities 1–6) (Koenig et al., 1988).

16. **Childbearing in the developing world is far more dangerous than use of oral contraceptives, IUDs, or condoms.**

16.a. An unplanned, unwanted pregnancy is 20 times riskier to the woman than use of any modern method of contraception (Rosenfield, cited in Starrs, 1987).

16.b. In Menoufia, Egypt, calculations from birth and death data, together with contraceptive use information, showed that one pregnancy and delivery was 48 times more risky than taking the pill for a year (Fortney et al., 1986).

16.c. The relative risks of contraceptive use versus pregnancy and childbearing can be heavily influenced by other risk factors, as well as by context. In England and Wales, for example, women over 40 who do not smoke have a lower risk of death from use of oral contraceptives than from pregnancy or childbirth. For women over 40 who do smoke, pill use is riskier than pregnancy and childbearing (Jain, 1977). The relative risks may be different in countries where medical services are underdeveloped (that is, where mortality risks of pregnancy and childbirth are high) (Segal, 1977).

Prenatal and Medical Care

17. **Prenatal care helps reduce death rates.**

17.a. Women who had never attended a prenatal care clinic died at 2.6 to 22 times the rate of clinic attenders in a number of studies reviewed by Zimicki (1989).

17.b. Though prenatal care provides an opportunity to predict in advance which women will have complications, such screening, even when done correctly, is often inaccurate (Winikoff et al., 1991). For example, in Zaire women who during screening were identified as being at high risk for obstructed labor were 9.2 times more likely to develop obstructed labor than were other women. However, they accounted for fewer than 33 percent of the women who later developed obstructed labor, and for every woman whose obstructed labor was correctly predicted, nine were treated as high risk but had perfectly normal deliveries (Maine et al., 1985).

17.c. Additionally, prenatal screening for maternal risk factors is often not done correctly. In the Côte d'Ivoire 73 percent of complications that should have been identified in prenatal visits (high blood pressure, anemia, narrow pelvis), were not (Maine et al., 1985).

18. **The existence of accessible medical facilities is critical. Approximately 15–20 percent of women who become pregnant develop serious complications that are hard to predict or prevent. Consequently, adequate and accessible medical care is essential for lowering maternal mortality.**

    18.a. The difference in maternal mortality between industrialized and least developed countries is of the order of 100- to 200-fold. In comparison, the difference in infant mortality between these two sets of countries is from 10- to 20-fold. In the past many of the improvements in infant and child mortality were attributable to the direct and indirect effects of socioeconomic development in general. This pattern of improvement in child survival has not been observed with respect to maternal mortality. Improvements in maternal health require functioning health systems, not merely community-level activities. They require skilled midwives, anesthesia, blood replacement, health centers, and hospitals. Between 10–15 percent of women require skilled assistance and facilities to handle the complications that arise during pregnancy and delivery. Without those skills and facilities, 10 percent of those women will die (Belsey, 1991).

    18.b. Incorrect or delayed treatment was an element in 11–47 percent of maternal deaths in studies in Colombia, Tanzania, Vietnam, and India. In Africa only about one-tenth of the women who need cesarean sections receive them (Maine et al., 1985). Of pregnant women in Addis Ababa who sought treatment for viral hepatitis, the majority were in or very near a coma by the time they arrived at the hospital (Kwast and Stevens, 1987). In the teaching hospital in Zaria, Nigeria, the family must buy drugs and sutures before a woman can be treated for obstructed labor. The waiting time between admission and surgery has increased from 3.5 to 7 hours in the last six years (Maine, no date).

    18.c. Rural health centers are usually the closest source of modern care for women experiencing difficult pregnancies or births. Unfortunately, staff of these centers are often unable to provide first aid for women who are hemorrhaging, in convulsions, or at risk of developing infection (Maine et al., 1985).

    18.d. Many of the smaller hospitals to which women are referred do not have the resources to maintain sterile conditions, perform cesarean sections, and provide blood transfusions, all of which are essential in the treatment of obstetric complications (Anon., 1987; Tazhib, 1983).

    18.e. With training, nurses and paramedical workers may be able to perform cesarean sections, administer prostaglandins, and do other procedures (Winikoff et al., 1991). In two hospitals in Zaire nurses performed 326 cesarean sections and laparotomies with only five deaths (White et al., 1987).

    18.f. Though many pregnant women rely solely on traditional birth attendants, TBAs often neglect prenatal care and hygiene. Training high proportions of active TBAs is difficult and expensive, and evidence on the success of such programs is mixed (Maine et al., 1985; Lettenmaier et al., 1988).

NOTES

1. 1983 estimates of ratios were developed for each subregion from local studies and other available information (Royston and Armstrong, 1989, pp. 30–35). UN estimates for the number of births in each region were then applied to obtain each subregion's number of maternal deaths. This analysis was updated for 1988.

2. In an ectopic pregnancy the fertilized egg implants in the wall of the fallopian tube

3. Hemorrhage can occur before or after birth and is often fatal unless treated by transfusion (Winikoff et al., 1991). Eclampsia is a condition of extremely high blood pressure, causing convulsions and, if untreated, stroke or heart failure. Obstructed labor causes several conditions—ruptured uterus, infection, exhaustion—any of which may be fatal. Infection can occur from nonsterile deliveries, premature rupture of the membranes, or long periods of obstructed labor. Fatal complications of abortion include infection and hemorrhage (Lettenmeier et al., 1988; Maine et al., 1985).

4. Evidence is limited because absolute numbers of deaths are usually small in any one study, and sample sizes are often too limited for detailed breakdowns by age and parity.

5. Numbers and rates of maternal deaths may fall by a proportion even greater than the reduction in pregnancies. The pregnancies that contraception prevents will likely occur disproportionately to women in high-risk groups, including women who opt for an unsafe abortion. Since these women have a higher risk of maternal death than the average woman, preventing their births will have a greater effect on maternal mortality than preventing births to other women. Whether the maternal mortality *ratio* will fall disproportionately is a separate question (see item 15).

REFERENCES

Adetoro, O.O. 1987. "Maternal mortality: A twelve-year study at the University of Ilorin Teaching Hospital, Ilorin, Nigeria." *International Journal of Gynaecology and Obstetrics* 25:93–98.

Anonymous. 1987. "Improving maternal care reduces mortality." *Network* 9(1):6–7.

Barford, D. and J. Parkes. 1977. "Maternal mortality: A survey of 118 maternal deaths and the avoidable factors." *South African Medical Journal* 51(4):101–105.

Belsey, M. 1991. "Priority issues in maternal and child health for the 1990s." Proceedings of the Demographic and Health Surveys World Conference, Washington, DC, August 5–7.

Blacker, J. 1987. "Health impacts of family planning." *Health Policy and Planning* 2(3):193–203.

Chen, L.C., M.C. Gesche, S. Ahmed, A.I. Chowdhury, and W. Mosley. 1974. "Maternal mortality in Bangladesh." *Studies in Family Planning* 5(11):334–341.

Costello, C. 1986. "Maternal and child health in rural Uganda: The role of nutrition." Doctoral dissertation in Demography: University of Pennsylvania.

Fauveau, V., M. Koenig, J. Chakraborty, and A. Chowdhury. 1988. "Causes of maternal mortality in rural Bangladesh." *Bulletin of the World Health Organization* 66(5):643–651.

Fortney, J. 1988. "Maternal mortality in Indonesia and Egypt." *International Journal of Gynaecology and Obstetrics* 26:21–32.

Fortney, J., I. Susanti, S. Gadalla, S. Saleh, S. Rogers, and M. Potts. 1986. "Reproductive mortality in two developing countries." *American Journal of Public Health* 76(2):134–138.

Graham, W., W. Brass, and R.W. Snow. 1989. "Estimating maternal mortality: The sisterhood method." *Studies in Family Planning* 20(3):125–135.

———. 1990. "Response" to James Trussell and Germán Rodriguez, "A note on the sisterhood estimator of maternal mortality." *Studies in Family Planning* 21(6):344–346.

Greenwood, A., B. Greenwood, A. Bradley, K. Williams, F. Shenton, S. Tulloch, P. Byass, and F. Oldfield. 1987. "A prospective survey of the outcome of pregnancy in a rural area of the Gambia." *Bulletin of the World Health Organization* 65(5): 635–643.

Harrison, K. 1987. "Maternal morbidity." *Network* 9(1):10–11.

Harrison, K. and L. Rossiter. 1985. "Childbearing, health, and social priorities: A survey of 22,774 consecutive hospital births in Zaria, Northern Nigeria." *British Journal of Obstetrics and Gynaecology* 92(Supplement 5):3–13.

Jain, A. 1977. "Mortality risk associated with the use of oral contraceptives." *Studies in Family Planning* 8(3):50–54.

Koenig, M., V. Fauveau, A. Chowdhury, J. Chakraborty, and M. Khan. 1988. "Maternal mortality in Matlab, Bangladesh: 1975–85." *Studies in Family Planning* 19(2):69–80.

Kwast, B.E. and J.A. Stevens. 1987. "Viral hepatitis as a major cause of maternal mortality in Addis Ababa, Ethiopia." *International Journal of Gynecology and Obstetrics* 25:99–106.

Lettenmaier, C., L. Liskin, C. Church, and J. Harris. 1988. "Mothers' lives matter: Maternal health in the community." *Population Reports* Series L, No. 7. Johns Hopkins University.

Maine, D. No date. *Safe Motherhood Programs: Options and Issues*. New York: Center for Population and Family Health, School of Public Health, Columbia University.

———.1988. "Maternal mortality: A problem whose time has come." *International Health News* 9(4):4.

Maine, D., R. McNamara, J. Wray, A. Farah, and M. Wallace. 1985. "Effects of fertility change on maternal and child survival." In *Population Growth and Reproduction in Sub-Saharan Africa: Technical Analyses of Fertility and its Consequences*. G.T.F. Acsadi, G. Johnson-Acsadi, and R.A. Bulatao, eds. Washington, DC: World Bank. Pp. 91–103.

Merchant, K. and R. Martorell. 1988. "Frequent reproductive cycling: Does it lead to nutritional depletion of mothers?" *Progress in Food and Nutrition Science* 12:339–369

Mhango, C., R. Rochat, and A. Arkutu. 1986. "Reproductive mortality in Lusaka, Zambia, 1982–1983." *Studies in Family Planning* 17(5):243–251.

National Academy of Sciences. 1989. *Contraception and Reproduction: Health Consequences for Women and Children in the Developing World*. Washington, DC: National Academy Press.

Rinehart, W., A. Kols, and S. Moore. 1984. "Healthier mothers and children through family planning." *Population Reports* Series J, no. 27. Johns Hopkins University.

Rochat, R. 1981. "Maternal mortality in the United States of America." *World Health Statistics Quarterly* 34(1):2–13.

Rooks, J. and B. Winikoff. 1990. "A reassessment of the concept of reproductive risk in maternity care and family planning services." Meeting proceedings from the Robert H. Ebert Program on Critical Issues in Reproductive Health and Population, The Population Council, New York, NY, February 12–13.

Royston, E. and S. Armstrong. 1989. *Preventing Maternal Deaths*. Geneva: World Health Organization.

Royston, E. and A. Lopez. 1987. "On the assessment of maternal mortality." *World Health Statistics Quarterly* 40:211–213.

Rutenberg, N. and J. Sullivan. 1991. "Direct and indirect estimates of maternal mortality from the sisterhood method." *Demographic and Health Surveys World Conference* Vol.III:1,669–1,696. Washington, DC: IRD/Macro International.

Segal, S. 1977. "Mortality risk with oral contraceptives: A comment." *Studies in Family Planning* 8(3):54.

Starrs, A. 1987. "Preventing the tragedy of maternal deaths: A report on the International Safe Motherhood Conference, Nairobi." Washington, DC: World Bank.

Tahzib, F. 1983. "Epidemiological determinants of vesico-vaginal fistulas." *British Journal of Obstetrics and Gynecology* 90(6): 387–391.

Trussell, J. and A. Pebley. 1984. "The potential impact of changes in fertility on infant, child, and maternal mortality." *Studies in Family Planning* 15(6):267–280.

Walker, G., D. Ashley, A. McCaw, and G. Bernard. 1985. "Maternal mortality in Jamaica: A confidential inquiry into all maternal deaths in Jamaica 1981–83." WHO FHE/PMM/85.9.10. WHO Interregional Meeting on Prevention of Maternal Mortality, Geneva, November 11–15.

White, S., R. Thorpe, and D. Maine. 1987. "Emergency obstetric surgery performed by nurses in Zaire." *Lancet* 2 (8,559):612–613.

Winikoff, B. 1987. "Family planning and the health of women and children." *Technology in Society* 9:415–438.

Winikoff, B. and M. Sullivan. 1987. "Assessing the role of family planning in reducing maternal mortality." *Studies in Family Planning* 18(3):128–143.

Winikoff, B. and M. Castle. 1988. "The maternal depletion syndrome: Clinical diagnosis or eco-demographic condition?" *Biology and Society* 5:163–170.

Winikoff, B., C. Carignan, E. Bernardik, and P. Semeraro. 1991. "Medical services to save mothers' lives: Feasible approaches to reducing maternal mortality." Programs Division *Working Papers* No. 4. New York: The Population Council.

World Health Organization (WHO). 1991. *Weekly Epidemiological Record* No. 47, 22 November. Geneva: WHO.

Zimicki, Susan. 1989. "The relationship between fertility and maternal mortality." In *Contraceptive Use and Controlled Fertility: Health Issues for Women and Children*. Allan Parnell, ed. Washington, DC: National Academy Press.

Chapter 12

CONTRACEPTIVE USE AND HEALTH

Contraceptives, while removing risks that attend pregnancy, also alter the user's risk of acquiring certain diseases or conditions. Evidence on the size of the benefits and risks associated with use of contraceptive methods comes primarily from the developed world. Effects for diseases prevalent only in less developed countries (schistosomiasis or malaria, for example) are not well-known.

ORAL CONTRACEPTIVES

Pelvic Inflammatory Disease and Reproductive Tract Infections

1. **Oral contraceptives reduce the risk of contracting pelvic inflammatory disease (PID) for women who have used them for at least one year.**

    1.a. Women who are currently using oral contraceptives and have used them for at least one year have a 40–50 percent lower risk of developing PID than do users of no method (Lee et al., 1989; Family Health International, 1986). In the United States in 1982 use of oral contraceptives prevented approximately 50,000 episodes of PID (Winikoff, 1987). Oral contraceptives are most effective against the more serious forms of PID and least effective against common reproductive tract infections, such as yeast infections (Hatcher et al., 1988). Use of oral contraceptives may increase the risk of vaginal candidiasis (Elias, 1991).

Breast Cancer

2. **Most studies show no overall increase in the risk of breast cancer for oral contraceptive (OC) users relative to nonusers. A few studies indicate that very specific subgroups of OC users experience increased risks. OC users face a reduced risk of benign breast disease.**

    2.a. A case-control study of Costa Rican women found no elevated risk of breast cancer for OC users compared with nonusers (Lee et al., 1987).

    2.b. OC users in the United States face no increased risk of breast cancer relative to nonusers, according to an analysis of case-control data from the Cancer and Steroid Hormone Study (CASH) of the Centers for Disease Control. Consideration of type of oral contraceptive did not change this result (Sattin et al., 1986).

    2.c. A further analysis of the CASH data revealed an increased risk of premenopausal breast cancer for women who experienced menarche before age 13, remained nulliparous, and had used OCs for eight or more years (relative risk of 3.8, compared with nonusers) (Stadel et al., 1988). Only a small number of cases were analyzed, but the results add to evidence from other studies that some subgroups of OC users may face higher risks of breast cancer than do nonusers (Holck, 1987; Anonymous, 1989).

    2.d. In developed countries current and recent users (within the past year) of oral contraceptives have a reduced risk of benign breast disease relative to noncontraceptors (Lee et al., 1989).

Endometrial and Ovarian Cancer

3. **Use of oral contraceptives significantly decreases the risk of endometrial and ovarian cancer relative to nonuse.**

    3.a. In eight published case-control studies, users of oral contraceptives have only 40–80 percent the risk of developing ovarian cancer that nonusers have. Protection appears to last for at least 10 years after discontinuation. Some studies demonstrate increased protection with duration of use (Holck, 1987).

    3.b. Women who use combined oral contraceptives—each tablet contains a mix of estrogen and progestogen—have a 50 percent lower risk of endometrial cancer than do nonusers, according to four case-control studies carried out in the United States (Holck, 1987). Additional studies carried out in other developed countries agree (World Health Organization, 1986b). Estrogen-only pills, however, appear to increase the risk of endometrial cancer (Holck, 1987).

Cervical Cancer

4. **The relationship between cervical cancer and use of hormonal contraceptives is difficult to analyze because it is confounded by numbers of sexual partners and frequency of Pap smears, which are related both to use of hormonal contraceptives and**

to risks of cervical cancer. The most careful studies show slightly increased risks of cervical cancer among users of hormonal contraceptives, but the differences are not always significant.

4.a. A World Health Organization case-control study that tried to control for numbers of sexual partners gave a relative risk of cervical cancer of 1.2 for OC users compared with nonusers (95 percent confidence interval of 1.0–1.4). These results are consistent with those of other well-designed studies, but epidemiologists remain unsure if they have adequately controlled for various confounding factors (Holck, 1987).

4.b. A case-control study of Costa Rican women found that OC users had no increased risk of developing invasive cervical cancer, relative to nonusers. For carcinoma in situ, however, risks for recent OC users were 1.6 relative to nonusers (95 percent confidence interval of 1.2–2.2) (Irwin et al., 1988).

Liver Cancer

5. Use of oral contraceptives significantly increases the risk of liver cancer, but liver cancer is so rare in most countries that the increase has little impact in terms of actual numbers of women with the disease.

5.a. A case-control study of women in the United Kingdom estimated the relative risk of liver cancer among OC users as 3.8 (95 percent confidence interval of 1.0 to 14.6). Use of the pill for eight years or more was associated with a 20 fold increase of death from liver cancer, compared with controls (Forman et al., 1986). These excess risks have little impact on the numbers of women with liver cancer, because the baseline risk of the disease is very low.

5.b. As yet no evidence on risks of liver cancer associated with use of oral contraceptives is available from the developing world (Holck, 1987). In countries where hepatitis B infection is common, use of oral contraceptives may increase the risk of liver cancer (Lee et al., 1989); the issue needs considerably more study. In some parts of the developing world the prevalence of hepatitis B virus may be 80 percent or more (Hatcher et al., 1988).

Cardiovascular Disease

6. Heart attacks and strokes occur more frequently among certain subgroups of OC users than among other OC users or nonusers.

6.a. Cardiovascular problems associated with use of OCs occur primarily to women over 35, women who smoke, and those with a prior history of high blood pressure, heart disease, or diabetes. Excess risk to younger women, especially those who do not smoke, is minimal (Hatcher et al., 1988).

6.b. Simulation studies provide information about risks of death from cardiovascular disease for women by age, smoking status, and OC use. Risks of death are greatest for women aged 40–44 who smoke more than 25 cigarettes per day and use the pill (208 deaths per 100,000 women). Fewer than 20 deaths occur per 100,000 women who are under 40 years old and smoke fewer than 25 cigarettes per day, even when they use the pill. Among women aged 20–44 who smoke more than 25 cigarettes per day, risks of death are eight to nine times higher for OC users than for nonusers. Among women aged 25–44 who use OCs, risks of death are 20 to 25 times higher for heavy smokers (25 or more cigarettes per day) than for nonsmokers (Kost et al., 1991).

6.c. In the United States women who take OCs for five years in their 30s lose 18 days of life expectancy, on average. Women over 45 lose an average of 80 days. Decreased life expectancy results from increased cardiovascular mortality (Fortney et al., 1986).

6.d. In the developing world many users of oral contraceptives are younger women trying to space their children. These are not the women for whom OC use raises the risk of heart disease (Gathinji, 1984).

Anemia and Glucose Tolerance

7. Oral contraceptives lower the risk of anemia.

7.a. Oral contraceptives help prevent anemia because they reduce the amount of blood lost through menstruation (Lee et al., 1989; Hatcher et al., 1988; Winikoff, 1987).

7.b. Substantial evidence shows that use of combined oral contraceptives (even low-dose OCs) is associated with decreases in glucose tolerance (WHO Task Force on Oral Contraceptives, unpublished data cited in World Health Organization, 1986b).

INJECTABLE CONTRACEPTIVES (DMPA)

Breast Cancer

8. There is little evidence to suggest a link between injectable contraception and breast cancer.

8.a. World Health Organization studies of women

in Kenya, Mexico, and Thailand, found no increased risk of breast cancer for women using injectable contraceptives (DMPA). The relative risk for DMPA users was 1.0 (95 percent confidence interval of 0.7 to 1.5). Risks did not change with increased duration of use (World Health Organization, 1986a).

8.b. A much smaller analysis in Costa Rica found that DMPA users had a relative risk of breast cancer of 2.6 compared with nonusers (95 percent confidence interval of 1.4 to 4.7). An elevated risk existed even for women who had used DMPA for less than one year. Because of the small number of cases and the lack of a dose-response relationship, the authors of this study warn that their results are inconclusive (Lee et al., 1987).

Endometrial and Ovarian Cancer

9. **Use of injectable contraceptives appears to reduce the risk of ovarian and endometrial cancer, but results are tentative because adequate data are scarce.**

9.a. The relative risk of endometrial cancer among users of DMPA, compared to controls, is estimated at .3 (95 percent confidence interval of 0.04 to 2.4) by the World Health Organization, using data from Kenya, Mexico, and Thailand. This estimate is tentative because very few cases were available for analysis. Nevertheless, the estimate, along with indirect evidence from endometrial biopsy studies and other sources, suggests that DMPA use is negatively associated with the risk of endometrial cancer (World Health Organization, 1986b; Holck, 1987).

9.b. The World Health Organization estimates the relative risk of ovarian cancer for DMPA users as 0.7, compared to nonusers (95 percent confidence intervals of 0.3 to 1.7). Again, the figure is tentative, but it suggests a negative relationship between DMPA use and risk of ovarian cancer (World Health Organization, 1986b).

Cervical Cancer

10. **DMPA use appears to have no effect on risks of cervical cancer.**

10.a. DMPA use does not appear to significantly raise the risk of cervical cancer, according to data collected by the World Health Organization in three developing countries. The estimated relative risk was 1.2 (confidence interval of 0.9 to 1.5) for DMPA users as opposed to nonusers (World Health Organization, 1986b).

Liver Cancer

11. **DMPA use does not appear to increase the risk of liver cancer.**

11.a. A World Health Organization analysis of data from Kenya, Mexico, and Thailand revealed no evidence of altered risk of liver cancer among users of DMPA (World Health Organization, 1986b).

Blood Composition

12. **Use of DMPA positively affects iron levels, while it has no effect on several other aspects of blood composition.**

12.a. Undernourished lactating women in Hyderabad, India showed a significant increase in their serum iron level after use of DMPA for one year (World Health Organization, 1986b).

12.b. Undernourished lactating women in the cities of Bombay and Hyderabad (India) and Chiang Mai (Thailand) experienced no change in liver function or in levels of serum protein, albumin, hemoglobin, or triglycerides after one year of DMPA use (data are from a longitudinal analysis conducted in family planning clinics in these cities by the World Health Organization, 1986b.)

12.c. DMPA users in the WHO study experienced no change in glucose tolerance and, in Bombay and Chiang Mai, a decrease in serum cholesterol levels (World Health Organization, 1986b).

NORPLANT®

Hemoglobin

13. **Use of NORPLANT® may increase blood levels of hemoglobin.**

13.a. Preliminary evidence from trials of NORPLANT® implants in six countries show that hemoglobin levels of continuing users rise slightly, despite intermittent bleeding and spotting (Sivin, 1988).

Procedural Complications of Insertion

14. **The medical procedure for inserting NORPLANT® is simple but carries some risk.**

14.a. NORPLANT® implantation carries slight risks of infection, expulsion, or local reaction. A study of

2,674 NORPLANT® acceptors in seven countries found one-year incidence rates of 0.8 percent for infection, 0.4 percent for expulsion, and 4.7 percent for a local reaction (pain or itching). Only three women expelled a capsule without prior evidence of infection, while 40 percent of the infections resulted in an expulsion. One-third of the infections and two-thirds of the expulsions occurred more than one month after implantation of the capsules, indicating that a follow-up period of several months may be necessary (Klavon and Grubb, 1989).

Ectopic Pregnancy

15. **NORPLANT® is associated with a decreased risk of ectopic pregnancy.**

15.a. In Population Council studies submitted to the Federal Drug Administration, the ectopic pregnancy rate among NORPLANT® users was 1.3 per 1,000 woman-years, and this rate is used in the United States in NORPLANT® labelling. Ectopic pregnancy rates are expected to diminish as the proportion of acceptors using improved implant technology increases (Sivin, personal communication, 1993).

15.b. Multi-country trials sponsored by the Population Council's International Committee for Contraception Research yielded an ectopic pregnancy rate among NORPLANT® users of .28 per 1,000 woman-years. This figure is influenced by data from China, where the ectopic pregnancy rate was only .1 per 1,000 woman-years (Sivin, 1988).

15.c. When NORPLANT® fails, the risk of ectopic pregnancy is increased. However, since NORPLANT® fails less than 1 percent of the time, the absolute risk of ectopic pregnancy is less with NORPLANT® than for women using IUDs or not contracepting at all.

INTRAUTERINE DEVICES

Reproductive Tract Infection and Pelvic Inflammatory Disease

16. **Use of an IUD alters a woman's risk of contracting a reproductive tract infection that could then lead to pelvic inflammatory disease (PID) or other serious outcomes (cervical cancer, systemic infection, increased risk of ectopic pregnancy, or HIV infection).**

16.a. Several studies and secondary analyses indicate that the risk of pelvic infection occurs primarily in the first four months after insertion (because of infection of the endometrial cavity at the time of insertion) and to women exposed to sexually transmitted diseases (Elias, 1991; Potts et al., 1991; Mishell, 1975; Treiman and Liskin, 1988). The risk of PID for women who are in a mutually monogamous sexual relationship is probably not increased by IUD use (Lee et al., 1989). Though these findings are encouraging, the difficulties of providing safe IUD insertions in resource-poor settings (where it may be hard to identify women with or exposed to sexually transmitted diseases) should not be ignored (Winikoff et al., 1993).

16.b. In Matlab, Bangladesh 68 percent of 472 symptomatic women were confirmed to have vaginal, cervical, or pelvic infection. Twenty-two percent of users of IUDs (and 24 percent of tubectomy users) were infected. Women using these methods were seven times more likely to be infected than were women who were not contracepting (Wasserheit et al., 1989).

Anemia and Blood Loss

17. **IUDs alter various indicators of nutritional status and metabolic functions.**

17.a. Nonhormonal IUDs increase the amount of blood lost during menstruation, because blood flow is heavier and bleeding lasts longer. Increased blood loss and lowered hemoglobin levels are most likely to occur during the first two years of use, after which they return to original levels (Andrade et al., 1988; Sivin et al., 1991). Greater loss of blood heightens the risk of anemia, which is a problem in developing countries, where anemia is already prevalent (Hatcher et al., 1988).

Insertion Procedure

18. **One major risk associated with IUD insertion is perforation of the uterus.**

18.a. Perforation of the uterus probably occurs in about one of 2,500 IUD insertions, though the exact frequency is unknown and some perforations are probably undetected. Risk of perforation increases if insertion occurs within two months of childbirth (Hatcher et al., 1988).

Tubal Infertility and Spontaneous Abortion

19. **Use of IUDs is associated indirectly with heightened risk of tubal infertility. For pregnant women**

who do not remove the IUD, there is a risk of spontaneous abortion.

19.a. Because IUD use increases the risk of developing PID for some women, IUDs are indirectly associated with increased risk of tubal infertility (Lee et al., 1989).

19.b. The annual failure rate of IUDs is only 1 percent or 2 percent, but if a woman does become pregnant and her IUD is left in, the chance of a spontaneous abortion is 50 percent. Early removal of the IUD reduces the chance to 25 percent (Lee et al., 1989).

Ectopic Pregnancy

20. IUDs are associated with a decreased risk of ectopic pregnancy.

20.a. Most IUDs protect against ectopic pregnancies. Users of IUDs with 200 mm^2 of copper had an ectopic pregnancy rate four-tenths that of noncontraceptors in the United States during 1970–78. For users of IUDs with 350mm^2 of copper or IUDs releasing 20mcg/day levonorgestrel, the ectopic pregnancy rate was one-tenth that of noncontraceptors. However, users of progesterone-releasing IUDs had ectopic pregnancy rates that were 50–80 percent above those of US noncontraceptors (1970–78) (Sivin, 1991).

In general, the IUD prevents more intrauterine pregnancies than ectopic pregnancies, so the *ratio* of ectopic to intrauterine pregnancies is greater among IUD users than among users of other methods (Hatcher et al., 1988).

FEMALE STERILIZATION

Procedural Complications

21. Surgical procedures carry risks of complications. Most complications of female sterilization are not serious, but occasionally there are grave outcomes.

21.a. Minor complications associated with sterilization include light hemorrhage, infection, and uterine perforation. A multinational study conducted by the World Health Organization reported that minor complications occur in 6–11 percent of sterilization procedures (Lee et al., 1989). A study in Matlab, Bangladesh indicated that among women showing symptoms of infection, those who had received a tubectomy were considerably more likely than noncontraceptors to be confirmed as infected (see 16.b.) (Wasserheit et al., 1989).

21.b. Serious complications from sterilization occur in only about 2 percent of the cases and include perforation of blood vessels or injury to the gastrointestinal tract and bowel injury. Risks of serious complications are doubled by obesity, lung disease, diabetes, or a history of PID (Lee et al., 1989).

21.c. Death resulting from sterilization procedures occurs very infrequently. Death-to-case rates for tubectomy were 19.3 per 100,000 operations in Bangladesh, according to a retrospective study of sterilizations taking place in 1979 and 1980. The most common causes of death were complications of anesthesia, tetanus, and hemorrhage. Though the sterilization procedure may carry some risk, of 100,000 operations performed, an estimated 1,015 women are saved from dying in pregnancy and childbirth at some time during the remainder of their reproductive span (Grimes et al., 1982).

Ectopic Pregnancy

22. Female sterilization so rarely fails that the associated risk of ectopic pregnancy is extremely low.

22.a. When sterilization fails, the risk of ectopic pregnancy is increased. However, since sterilization fails less than 1 percent of the time, the absolute risk of ectopic pregnancy is less for sterilized women than for women using IUDs or not contracepting at all (Lee et al., 1989; Hatcher et al., 1988).

MALE STERILIZATION

Procedural Complications

23. As a minor surgical procedure, vasectomy produces few complications.

23.a. Any complications usually subside within one or two weeks. Hematomas (a collection of blood under the skin) usually occur in less than 1 percent of cases, and infection in less than 2 percent of cases, though the proportion is higher when surgical routines are careless or where excessive physical activity following the procedure encourages hematomas. Together, infection and hematomas occur in fewer than 3 percent of cases (Liskin et al., 1983).

23.b. No-scalpel vasectomy (NSV) has even fewer side effects than does conventional vasectomy. (Instead of an incision to enter the scrotum, with NSV a tiny puncture is made in the scrotal skin and widened enough to draw out the vas, which is then blocked by one of the usual methods.) Over 9 million NSVs have been performed in China, and the procedure is being performed increasingly in other countries including the US. Numerous studies report fewer complications for NSV than for conventional vasectomy, and a five-country randomized clinical trial (preliminary results) of almost 1,000 men shows significantly fewer complications and complaints with NSV than with the traditional procedure (Family Health International, 1991, cited in Liskin et al., 1992).

23.c. Long-term safety after vasectomy is excellent. Over 15 major studies show that vasectomized men are not at greater risk of any clinical diseases than are other men (Liskin et al., 1992). In the largest study done so far, 22,000 vasectomized men had similar or lower rates of 98 diseases than did controls (Massey et al., 1984). Only genitourinary tract infections or inflammations (up to two years after vasectomy) showed elevated rates, and these are minor and easily treated. A few studies linking vasectomy to prostate or testicular cancer are contradicted by other, more carefully designed studies; a review of available evidence by experts convened by the World Health Organization found no causal connection between vasectomy and cancer (Liskin et al., 1992).

CONDOMS AND SPERMICIDES

HIV Infection

24. Use of condoms and spermicides can lessen the risk of HIV infection. Use of these methods is the only recourse for protection apart from abstinence, mutual monogamy, or restraint in sexual activity (avoiding direct contact with the genital area and body fluids).

24.a. In a study of 546 prostitutes in the United States, 11 percent of the 524 prostitutes who reported having unprotected vaginal intercourse were HIV positive. None of the 22 prostitutes whose clients had used condoms in every episode of vaginal intercourse was HIV positive (Centers for Disease Control, 1987).

24.b. In a study in Zaire, 34 percent of the 77 prostitutes who reported that under half of their clients used condoms were HIV positive, while none of the 8 prostitutes who reported that over half of their clients used condoms was infected (Mann et al., 1987).

24.c. Among married couples in the US in which one partner had AIDS, the relative risk of the other partner testing HIV positive was 0.1 to 0.2 for couples who used condoms, compared with couples who did not (couples were followed for 12–36 months). Among couples using condoms, 17 percent of the uninfected partners eventually tested positive for HIV, while 82 percent of the nonusers did so (Fischl et al., 1987).

24.d. Several laboratory studies have demonstrated that HIV cannot pass through latex and synthetic skin condoms (Feldblum and Fortney, 1988), but it does appear to pass through some natural skin condoms (Centers for Disease Control, 1988).

24.e. Additionally, nonoxynol-9, the active ingredient used in many commercial spermicides and in contraceptive sponges, inactivates HIV (Feldblum and Fortney, 1988), although it is not clear that use of spermicides in the anal canal can prevent transmission of HIV (Centers for Disease Control, 1988).

24.f. Condoms do not provide adequate protection against infections spread from lesions rather than fluids, since condoms do not cover all the skin areas that might be infectious or infectable (Centers for Disease Control, 1988).

Reproductive Tract Infections and Pelvic Inflammatory Disease

25. Use of condoms and spermicides lowers the risk of reproductive tract infections that can lead to pelvic inflammatory disease (PID) or other serious outcomes (cervical cancer, systemic infection, increased risk of ectopic pregnancy, or HIV infection).

25.a. Barrier methods of contraception, especially when used with spermicides, can protect women from a variety of sexually transmitted diseases that may lead to reproductive tract infections and PID (Kols et al., 1982; Winikoff, 1987).

25.b. Laboratory studies indicate that latex condoms are impermeable to the herpes simplex virus, cytomegalovirus, hepatitis B, *Chlamydia trachomatis* (responsible for yeast infection), and *Neisseria gonorrhoea*. Both cross-sectional and case-control studies reveal lower frequencies of gonorrhea, ureaplasma infection, pelvic inflammatory disease, and cervical cancer among condom users than among nonusers (Centers for Disease Control, 1988).

REFERENCES

Andrade, A.T.L. et al. 1988. "Consequences of uterine blood loss caused by various intrauterine contraceptive devices in South American women." *Contraception.* 38(1):1–18.

Anonymous. 1989. "FDA reviews new reports on OC use and breast cancer risk." *Outlook* March:6–8.

Centers for Disease Control. 1987. "Antibody to human immunodeficiency virus." *Morbidity and Mortality Weekly Report* 36:157–161.

———. 1988. "Condoms for the prevention of sexually transmitted diseases." *Morbidity and Mortality Weekly Report* 37(9):133–137.

Elias, C. 1991. "Sexually transmitted diseases and the reproductive health of women in developing countries." *Programs Division Working Papers,* No. 5. New York: The Population Council.

Family Health International. 1986. "Risks and benefits of the pill." *Network* 7(4):4–5.

———. 1991. "Comparative Trial of NSV and Standard Incision Approaches to Vasectomy: Early Follow-up Complications and Complaints." Research Triangle Park, North Carolina: FHI, August 12.

Feldblum, P.J. and J.A. Fortney. 1988. "Condoms, spermicides, and the transmission of human immunodeficiency virus: A review of the literature." *American Journal of Public Health* 78(1):52–54.

Fischl, M., G. Dickinson, and G. Scott. 1987. "Evaluation of heterosexual partners, children, and household contacts of adults with AIDS." *Journal of the American Medical Association* 257:640–644.

Forman, D., T.J. Vincent, and R. Doll. 1986. "Cancer of the liver and the use of oral contraceptives." *British Medical Journal* 292:1,357–1,361.

Fortney, J., J. Harper, and M. Potts. 1986. "Oral contraceptives and life expectancy." *Studies in Family Planning* 17(3):117–125.

Gathinji, I. 1984. "Oral contraceptives." In *Reproductive Health.* J.K.G. Mati, O.A. Ladipo, R. Burkman, R. Magarick, and D. Huber, eds. Baltimore, MD: Johns Hopkins Program for International Education in Gynecology and Obstetrics.

Grimes, D.A., H.B. Peterson, M.J. Rosenberg, J.I. Fishburne, R.W. Rochat, A.R. Khan, and R. Islam. 1982. "Sterilization-attributable deaths in Bangladesh." *International Journal of Gynecology and Obstetrics* 20:149–154.

Hatcher, R.A., F. Guest, F. Stewart, G.K. Stewart, J. Trussell, S.C. Bowen, and W. Cates. 1988. *Contraceptive Technology 1988–1989.* New York: Irvington.

Holck, S. 1987. "Hormonal contraceptives and the risk of cancer." *World Health Statistical Quarterly* 40:225–232.

Irwin, K., L. Rosero-Bixby, M.W. Oberle, N.C. Lee, A.S. Whatley, J.A. Fortney, and M.G. Bonhomme. 1988. "Oral contraceptives and cervical cancer risk in Costa Rica: Detection bias or causal association?" *Journal of the American Medical Association* 259(1):59–64.

Klavon, S. and G. Grubb. 1989. "Insertion site complications during the first year of NORPLANT use." *Contraception* 41(1):27–37.

Kols, A. et al. 1982. "Oral contraceptives in the 1980s." *Population Reports* Series A-6, 10(3):189–222.

Kost, K., J. Forrest, and S. Harlap. 1991. "Comparing the health risks and benefits of contraceptive choices." *Family Planning Perspectives* 23(2):54–61.

Lee, N., L. Rosero-Bixby, M.W. Oberle, C. Grimaldo, A.S. Whatley, and E.Z. Rovira. 1987. "A case-control study of breast cancer and hormonal contraception in Costa Rica." *Journal of the National Cancer Institute* 79(6):1,247–1,254.

Lee, N., H. Peterson, and S. Chu. 1989. "Health effects of contraception." In *Contraceptive Use and Controlled Fertility: Health Issues for Women and Children.* A.M. Parnell, ed. Washington DC: National Academy Press.

Liskin, L., J.M. Pile, and W.F. Quillin. 1983. "Vasectomy: Safe and simple." *Population Reports* 11(5) Series D, No. 4.

Liskin, L., E. Benoit, and R. Blackburn. 1992. "Vasectomy: New opportunities." *Population Reports* 20(1) Series D, No. 5.

Mann, J., T. Quinn, and P. Plot. 1987. "Condom use and HIV infection among prostitutes in Zaire." *New England Journal of Medicine* 316:345.

Massey, F.J. Jr., G.S. Bernstein, and W.M. O'Fallon. 1984. "Vasectomy and health: Results from a large cohort study." *Journal of the American Medical Association* 252(8):1,023–1,029.

Mishell, D.R. 1975. "The clinic factor in evaluating IUDs." In *Analysis of Intrauterine Contraception.* F. Hefnawi, and S.J. Segal, eds. New York: American Elsevier.

Potts, M., C.B. Champion, M. Kozuh-Novak, and F. Alvarez-Sanchez. 1991. "IUDs and PID: A comparative trial of strings versus stringless devices." *Advances in Contraception* 7:231–240.

Sattin, R.W., G.L. Rubin, P.A. Wingo, L.A. Webster, and H.W. Ory. 1986. "Oral-contraceptive use and the risk of breast cancer. The Cancer and Steroid Hormone Study of the Centers for Disease Control and the National Institute of Child Health and Human Development." *New England Journal of Medicine* 315(7):405–411.

Sivin, I. 1988. "International experience with NORPLANT® and NORPLANT®-2 contraceptives." *Studies in Family Planning* 19(2):81–94.

———. 1991. "Dose- and age-dependent ectopic pregnancy risks with intrauterine contraception." *Obstetrics and Gynecology* 78(2):291–298.

———. 1993. Personal communication.

Sivin, I. et al. 1991. "Prolonged intrauterine contraception: A seven-year randomized study of the levonorgestrel 20 mcg/day (LNg 20) and the Copper T380 Ag IUDs." *Contraception* 44(5):473–480.

Stadel, B.V. 1988. "Oral contraceptives and premenopausal breast cancer in nulliparous women." *Contraception* 38(3):287–299.

Treiman, K. and L. Liskin. 1988. "IUDs—A new look." *Population Reports.* Series B-5. 16(1):1–32.

Wasserheit, J., J.R. Harris, J. Chakraborty, B.A. Kay, and K.J. Mason. 1989. "Reproductive tract infections in a family planning program in rural Bangladesh." *Studies in Family Planning* 20(2):69–80.

Winikoff, B. 1987. "Family planning and the health of women and children." *Technology in Science* 9:415–438.

Winikoff, B., C. Elias, and K. Beattie. 1993. "Special issues in resource-poor settings." In *A New Look at IUDs: Advancing Contraceptive Choices.* C.W. Bardin and D.R. Mishell, Jr., eds. Boston: Butterworth-Heinemann. Forthcoming.

World Health Organization. 1986a. "Metabolic side-effects of injectable depot-medroxyprogesterone acetate, 150 mg three-monthly, in undernourished lactating women." *Bulletin of the World Health Organization* 64(4):587–594.

———. 1986b. "Depot-medroxyprogesterone acetate (DMPA) and cancer: Memorandum from a WHO Meeting." *Bulletin of the World Health Organization* 64(3):375–382.

Index

A

Abortion, induced, 63–74
    averted by sterilization, 59
    birth rate decline and, 65, 66
    characteristics of abortion clients, 64–65
        age, 64–65
        marital status, 64
        parity, 64–65
    complications, 69–71
        cervical laceration, 70
        in developing countries, 69–70
        hemorrhage, 70
        septic abortion, 70
        uterine perforation, 70
    contraceptive use, as backup for, 66
    contraceptive use combined with abortion by women highly motivated to control their fertility, 66
    by curettage, 72
    demographics of, 65–67
    by dilation and evacuation, 73
    incidence of, 63–64
        hospital data, 63–64
        regionally, 63, 64
        statistical frequency, 63
    increase of contraceptive use after, 67
    legality of, 63, 67–69
        as indicator of availability, 67
        mortality, effect on, 69, 70–71
        recent legislation, 67–69
        variation from country to country, 67, 68
    by medical induction, 73
    by menstrual regulation, 72
    modern methods of, 72–73
    mortality associated with, 69–70
        liberalization of abortion laws, effect of, 69, 70–71
        safety as surgical procedure, 69
        from septic abortion, 70
        U.S. statistics on reported maternal deaths, 69
    postpartum programs, effect on, 37
    ratio of abortions to prevented births, 66
    with RU486, 72–73
    stage of fertility transition and abortion rates, 65
    traditional methods of, 71–72
        traditional practitioners, 71–72
        types of, 71
    by vacuum aspiration, 72
    see also Spontaneous abortion
Abstinence, periodic:
    continuation rates, 49
    failure rates, 50
Accidental pregnancy, contraceptive method chosen after, 54
Africa, fertility trends in, 8
Age:
    contraceptive continuation and, 52
    failure of contraceptive method and, 53
    induced abortion and, 64–65
    maternal mortality and, 84, 85
    sterilization and, 59, 61
Anemia, 91, 93
Asia, fertility trends in, 8

B

Barrier contraceptive methods:
    condoms, *see* Condoms
    sexually transmitted diseases, and infant and child mortality, 80
Blood composition and DMPA, 92
Breast cancer, 90, 91–92
Breastfeeding as contraceptive method, 37–38

C

Cardiovascular disease, 91
Cervical cancer, 90–91, 92
Cervical laceration from induced abortion, 70
Charges and payments associated with provision of family planning services, 40–47
    effect of charges on contraceptive use, 44–46
        cost as barrier to contraceptive use, 46
        lowering of prices, demand and, 45
        price sensitivity of more effective methods, 46
        pros and cons of charges for contraceptive supplies, 44–45
        small charges versus free contraceptives, 45–46
    effect of payments on contraceptive use, 43–44
        contributory factors along with desire to limit family size, 43
        men versus women, sterilization acceptance by, 43–44
        motivators, payments to, 44
        poor versus rich as acceptors, 43
        prevalence levels of methods for which rewards are offered, 43
        sterilization acceptance by men versus women, 43–44
    structure of charges and payments, 40, 41
    types of payments, 40–43
        community-focused incentive schemes, 42
        non-cash incentives and disincentives, 42–43
        one-time cash award for sterilization or IUD, 40
        payment to motivators or providers on per-case basis, 41–42
Child mortality, *see* Contraception, fertility patterns, and infant and child mortality
China, family planning programs in, 13
Community-based distribution (CBD), 22–26
    charges for services, 24
    coverage, 22
    distribution strategies, 23–24
    effort levels, 22–23
    outcomes, 23
    providers, 22
    supervision, 25–26
    training, 25
Condoms:
    continuation rates, 49
    discontinuation, reasons for, 51
    failure rates, 50
    health issues, 95
Continuation of contraceptive use, *see* Contraceptive continuation and effectiveness
Contraception, fertility patterns, and infant and child

mortality, 75–81
  bivariate relationships, 75–76
    birth order, 75–76
    births to older women, 57
    preceding interval length, 76
    teenage mothers, 75
  changes in distribution of births as fertility declines, 78–79
  changes in infant and child mortality rates due to changes in pace and ages at which childbearing occurs, 79
  multivariate relationships, 75, 76–78
    biodemographic factors, 76
    births to teenagers, 76, 78
    children of older women, 76–77
    combinations of risk factors, 77–78
    first births, 77
    higher order births, 77
    previous birth intervals, 77
    socioeconomic factors, 76
    subsequent birth intervals, 77
  reduction in infant and child mortality with contraceptive use, 75
  sexually transmitted diseases, barrier methods and, 80
  unwanted births, 79–80
Contraceptive continuation and effectiveness, 48–56
  aggregated continuation and failure rates, 48
  contraceptive continuation rates, 48–49
    condoms, 49
    injectables, 48
    IUDs, 48, 49
    longer-term data, 49
    NORPLANT®, 49
    oral contraceptives, 48
    periodic abstinence, 49
  contraceptive failure rates, 49–50
    condoms, 50
    injectables, 50
    IUDs, 50
    NORPLANT®, 50
    oral contraceptives, 49–50
    periodic abstinence, 50
    sterilization, 49
  correlates of continuation, 50–53
    age, 52
    desire for more children, 53
    education, 53
    by method, 50–52
    parity, 52
    personal characteristics, 52–53
    side effects, medical reasons, and failures, 50–52
    son preference, 52–53
  correlates of failure, 53–54
    accidental pregnancy, method after, 54
    by age, 53
    by duration of use, 54
    by education, 53–54
    by method, 53
    by parity, 53
    programs offering a variety of method choices, 54
    by residence, 53–54
  information on, sources of, 48
  life-table techniques for calculating, 48
  prevalence sensitivity to continuation rates, 48
Contraceptive social marketing (CSM), 27–33
  cost-effectiveness, 31–32
  coverage, 27
  effort levels, 27
  management features, 30
  objectives, 27
  overview, 27
  pricing, 30–31
  promotional efforts, 31
  sales and couple-years of protection, 27–29
  substitution for other supply sources, 30
Contraceptive use:
  abortion as backup to, 66
  combined with abortion by highly motivated women, 66
  fertility patterns, and infant and child mortality, *see* Contraception, fertility patterns, and infant and child mortality
  health and, *see* Health and contraceptive use
  increase of, after abortion, 67
  maternal morbidity/mortality and, 85–86
  prevalence, *see* Prevalence of contraceptive use
  private sector's role as source of supply for contraceptives, 16–17
  as program supplied in developing world, 15–16, 17
Couple-years of protection, sales of contraceptives through social marketing and, 27–29
Curettage, abortion by, 72

D

Delivery of contraceptive, *see* Suppliers of contraceptives
Demographics:
  of abortion, 65–67
  sterilization, demographic effects of, 59
Desire for more children, contraceptive continuation and, 53
Dilation and evacuation, abortion by, 73
Distribution, community-based, *see* Community-based distribution
DMPA, 91–92

E

Ectopic pregnancy, 93, 94
Education:
  contraceptive continuation and, 53
  failure of contraceptive method and, 53–54
Effectiveness of contraceptive method, *see* Contraceptive continuation and effectiveness
Endometrial cancer, 90, 92

F

Failure of contraceptives, *see* Contraceptive continuation and effectiveness
Family planning programs, large-scale, *see* Large-scale family planning programs
Family size, sterilization and, 59
Fertility patterns:
  fertility levels and family planning program effort, 19, 20

prevalence of contraceptive use and, *see* Prevalence of contraceptive use and fertility patterns

G

Glucose tolerance and oral contraceptives, 91

H

Health and contraceptive use, 90–96
    condoms and spermicides, 95
    injectable contraceptives (DMPA), 91–92
        blood composition, 92
        breast cancer, 91–92
        cervical cancer, 92
        endometrial cancer, 92
        liver cancer, 92
        ovarian cancer, 92
    IUDs, 93–94
        anemia and blood loss, 93
        ectopic pregnancy, 94
        insertion procedure, 93
        pelvic inflammatory disease, 93
        reproductive tract infection, 93
        spontaneous abortion, 93–94
        tubal infertility, 93
    NORPLANT®, 92–93
        ectopic pregnancy, 93
        hemoglobin, 92
        procedural complications of insertion, 92–93
    oral contraceptives, 90–91
        anemia, 91
        breast cancer, 90
        cardiovascular disease, 91
        cervical cancer, 90–91
        endometrial cancer, 90
        glucose tolerance, 91
        liver cancer, 91
        ovarian cancer, 90
    sterilization, 94–95
Hemoglobin levels and NORPLANT®, 92
Hemorrhage from induced abortion, 70
HIV infection, 95

I

India, family planning programs in, 13
Induced abortion, *see* Abortion, induced
Infant mortality, *see* Contraception, fertility patterns, and infant and child mortality
Injectables:
    continuation rates for, 48
    discontinuation, reasons for, 50, 51
    failure rates, 50
    health and, *see* Health and contraceptive use, injectable contraceptives (DMPA)
Intrauterine devices, *see* IUDs
IUDs:
    continuation rates, 48, 49
    discontinuation, reasons for, 50–51, 52
    failure rates, 50
    health and, *see* Health and contraceptive use, IUDs
    one–time cash award for acceptors of, 40

L

Large–scale family planning programs, 13–21
    in China, 13
    contraceptive use in developing world as program supplied, 15–16, 17
    coverage of the population for each function, 13
    fertility levels and program effort, 19, 20
    formal barriers constricting, 15
    improvement in program efforts since 1972, 13
    in India, 13
    individual countries with weak programs, 13
    level of country's development and program effort, 19–20
    long–acting methods, programs that encourage adoption of, 18
    majority of people living in countries with strong, 13
    modes of delivery, 13
    outreach items, differences between strong and weak programs on, 13–15
    prevalence and influence of contraceptive effectiveness on fertility, 19
    prevalence of use and number of methods available, 17–18
    principal functions of, 13
    private sector's role as source of supply for contraceptive users, 16–17
    Program Effort Scores, 13, 15
        itemization of, 14
    ratings of program effort, 13
    selectivity of programs in their efforts, 13
    socioeconomic setting:
        relationship of contraceptive prevalence to program effort, 19
        weakening of socioeconomic differentials under strong programs, 20
        weaker programs, selective improvement of, 15
Latin America, fertility trends in, 8
Liver cancer, 91, 92

M

Marital status, induced abortion and, 64
Maternal morbidity/mortality, 82–89
    causes of maternal mortality, 83–84
        direct, 83–84
        indirect, 84
    children left behind after death of mother, 83
    data and measurement, 82
    definitions, 82
    extent of maternal morbidity, 83
    extent of maternal mortality, 82–83
    interventions, 85–87
        contraceptive use, 85–86
        medical care, 87
        prenatal care, 86–87
    nutritional status, effect of childbearing on, 83
    overview, 82

reproductive risk factors, 84–85
   age, 84
   birth intervals, 85
   combination of age and parity, 85
   parity/gravidity, 84–85
Menstrual regulation, abortion by, 72
Morbidity, maternal, see Maternal morbidity/mortality
Mortality:
   abortion, see Abortion, induced
   infant and child, see Contraception, fertility patterns, and infant and child mortality
   maternal, see Maternal morbidity/mortality

N

NORPLANT®:
   continuation rates for, 48
   discontinuation, reasons for, 50, 51
   failure rates for, 50
   health issues, 92–93
      ectopic pregnancy, 93
      hemoglobin, 92
      procedural complications of insertion, 92–93

O

Oral contraceptives:
   continuation rates, 48
   discontinuation, reasons for, 51, 52
   failure rates, 49–50
   health and, see Health and contraceptive use, oral contraceptives
Ovarian cancer, 90, 92

P

Parity:
   contraceptive continuation and, 52
   failure of contraceptive method and, 53
   induced abortion and, 64–65
   maternal mortality and, 84–85
Payments associated with provision of family planning services, see Charges and payments associated with provision of family planning services
Pelvic inflammatory disease, 93, 95
Periodic abstinence, see Abstinence, periodic
Pill, the, see Oral contraceptives
Postpartum programs, 34–39
   abortions, effects upon, 37
   advantages of, 34
   breastfeeding as contraceptive method, 37–38
   coverage and potential, 34–35
   current method recommendations, 36
   described, 34
   difference between actual and desired birth interval length, 36
   disadvantages of, 34
   interest in, 36–37
   overlap of contraceptive use and postpartum amenorrhea, 38–39
   unmet needs, 35–36

Prenatal care and maternal mortality, 86–87
Prevalence of contraceptive use:
   continuation rates and, 48
   fertility patterns and, see Prevalence of contraceptive use and fertility patterns
   influence of contraceptive effectiveness on fertility as related to, 19
   number of available methods and, 17–18
   socioeconomic setting and family planning program effort, 19
   sterilization, 57–58
      male versus female, 57–58, 59
Prevalence of contraceptive use and fertility patterns, 1–12
   fertility trends, 8–12
      in Africa, 8
      in Asia, 8
      crude birth rate and, 10
      in the developing world, by region, 2, 9
      in Latin America, 8
      life expectancy and, 10–11
      more recent declines and rate of decline, 11
      overall, 8
      pace of decline in last two five–year periods, 8
      subreplacement fertility, 11
      total fertility rate and net reproduction rate, 9–10
   method, prevalence by, 2–7
      countries and regions, 3–6
      modern versus traditional methods, 6–7
      most prevalent methods, 2–3
   personal characteristics, prevalence by, 7–8
   prevalence
      in largest countries, 1
      people living in countries with moderate to high, 1
   prevalence:
      countries, low level of prevalence in most, 1
      developing countries distributed by level of, 3
      in developing world, by region, 2, 4–5
      in the future, 1–2
      geographic patterns, variation in, 1
      by method, 2–7
      overview, 1
      by personal characteristics, 7–8
      sustained increases in prevalence, counties with, 1
      total fertility rate and, 1, 2, 6

R

Reproductive tract infection, 93, 95
Residence:
   failure of contraceptive method and, 53–54
   sterilization and, 59
Rhythm method, reasons for discontinuation of, 51
RU486, 72–73

S

Septic abortion, 70
Sexually transmitted diseases (STDs), 95
   barrier methods, and infant and child mortality, 80
   HIV infection, condoms and spermicides and, 95
Social marketing, contraceptive, see Contraceptive social marketing

Socioeconomic setting:
    infant and child mortality, multivariate relationships, 76
    large–scale family planning programs:
        relationship of contraceptive prevalence to program effort, 19
        weakening of socioeconomic differentials under strong programs, 20
    sterilization and, 59
Son preference and contraceptive continuation, 52–53
Spermicides, condoms, and health issues, 95
Spontaneous abortion, 93–94
Sterilization, 57–62
    advantages of, 57
    age and, 59, 61
    demographic effects of, 59–60
    disadvantages of, 57
    dynamics of, 58
    failure rates, 49
    legal aspects of, 60–62
    morbidity and mortality, 62
    number of living children and, 59
    one–time cash award for acceptors of, 40
    payments for, and acceptance by men versus women, 43–44
    personal characteristics of users, 59, 61
    prevalence of, 57–58
        male versus female sterilization, 57–58, 59
    psychological and social–psychological variables, 59
    residence and, 59
    socioeconomic status and, 59
Suppliers of contraceptives:
    private sector, 16–17
    social marketing, *see* Contraceptive social marketing

T

Teenagers:
    infant and child mortality, risk of, 76, 78
    maternal mortality, risk of, 84
Tubal infertility, 93
Tubectomy, *see* Sterilization

U

Uterine perforation from induced abortion, 70

V

Vacuum aspiration, abortion by, 72
Vasectomy, *see* Sterilization